How to lose fat and develop strong Abdominal Muscles with Simple Six Pack Training

By:
Joerg Weber
http://www.welchediaet.de

No matter if male or female, everyone wants a perfect body in order to be attractive. If you feel attractive your self-confidence will rise automatically.

We become racier and more secure, in essence adored by others. But this is not the only thing as we keep fit and also live healthier; our stamina increases and the concentration is improving. Just those things alone should be motivating for you. Shouldn't they?

This book will mainly talk about abdominal muscle s and six pack training Our abdominal muscle s represent a large area of our body.

It takes some discipline, motivation, the right kind of diet, and a strict exercise plan for a man to hear that sigh and „ What a guy!„ And for a woman to attract the desirable looks from men around her.

Following a brief overview what you can expect from this unique how-to manual.

Abdominal muscles
Abdominal Muscle Overview

Abdominal muscles are much more important than you may think. You have to understand how this muscle group is built in order to get a flat stomach, ripped abs or six pack abs. You should have some basic knowledge to make it easier to read and understand this book, and most important understand how important the right diet is together with the right work out plan.

For starters – everyone has abdominal muscle s, i.e. six pack abs. You don't believe it? Let me ask you: "Can you stand up, walk straight, sit and breathe? " Of course you can do all of this, because you have a hidden six pack.

Abdominal muscles are stabilizing the pelvis and spine, as well as carrying your organs.

If your abdominal muscle s are weak you may encounter back pain, and digestive problems since the muscles are too weak to support your inner organs.

Abdominal muscles are comprised of the following:

- Surface abdominal muscles
  o Diagonal abdominal muscles
    ▪ Outer oblique abdominal muscle (lat. musculus obliquus externus

      abdominis)
    ▪ Inner oblique abdominal muscle (lat. musculus obliquus internus

      abdominis)
    ▪ Transverse abdominal muscle (lat. musculus transversus abdominis)

  o Middle muscle group
    ▪ Straight abdominal muscle (lat. musculus rectus abdominis)
    ▪ Pyramid muscle (lat. musculus pyramidalis)

- Deep abdominal muscles
  o Square lumbar muscle (lat. musculus quadratus lumborum)

  o Large lumbar muscle (lat. musculus psoas major)

As you can see, abdominal muscles are rather complex. In the following chapters the muscles will be described in further detail.

The outer oblique abdominal muscle

The largest abdominal muscle of the stomach muscle group is the outer oblique abdominal muscle. He is situated on the surface of your abdominal muscles running from the outside of the fifth to the twelfth rib to the dam crest bone

The outer oblique abdominal muscle (lat. musculus obliquus externus abdominis) is an approximately 2.7 inch thick layer. It supports the straight abdominal muscle. You should work out this muscle not only because of aesthetic but also health reasons

The outer oblique abdominal muscle works together with the inner oblique abdominal muscle, and also supports the straight abdominal muscle while straightening out your upper body.

Additional functions of this muscle are rotating the torso to the opposite side, assisting in bending your torso forward, in raising the anterior pelvic ring, in bending the thorax towards the opposite side and assisting tightening your stomach.

The inner oblique abdominal muscle

The smallest among the side abdominal muscles is the inner oblique abdominal muscle (lat. Musculus obliquus internus abdominis) which is situated direct underneath the outer oblique abdominal muscle. It is a three sided approximately 0.4 inch thick muscle. The starting point of the inner oblique abdominal muscle is between the ninth and twelfth rib and has its origin at the inguinal ligament.

This muscle helps the torso to lift and carry heavy loads, and is important for breathing, i.e. exhaling, just like the outer oblique abdominal muscle. Further is also compresses the stomach, is used to stretch, incline, and bend the torso forward. The inner oblique abdominal muscle supports the straight abdominal muscle.

The transverse abdominal muscle

The transverse abdominal muscle (lat. musculus transversus abdominis) is the deepest layer of abdominal muscles and is situated underneath the oblique abdominal muscle. It stretches from the lower ribs, lumbar vertebrae and the lateral resolutions of the iliac crest to the tendon sheath of the straight abdominal muscle (rectus abdominis muscle). The waist is formed by the cross and oblique abdominal muscle

The transverse muscle is used to erect the pelvis in conjunction to the cross abdominal muscle. This muscle is responsible to rotate the torso, to exhale, and assists in compressing the stomach as well as lowering the rib cage.

The straight abdominal muscle

This abdominal muscle is called musculus rectus abdominis in Latin. This muscle is the actual six pack muscle and is the largest abdominal muscle. It is a large and flat muscle originating from the xiphoid of the sternum and runs all the way to the pelvic in two strips.

The straight muscle is important for bending and fixating the torso when you are carrying something. It is just as important to hold and lift the pelvis.

The Pyramid Muscle

The Pyramid muscle (lat. musculus pyramidalis) is important for marsupials. In 16 – 25% of all humans it can be missing. It is a rather insignificant muscle. He is one of the front central abdominal muscles and his shape is triangular.

The square loin muscle

The square loin muscle, in Latin musculus quadratus lumborum, is part of the deep abdominal muscles. It lies between the rear part of the dam crest and the 12th rib.

Its functions are the sideways tilt of the torso, stretching the lumbar spine, and assistance with exhalation.

The large loin muscle

The large loin muscle, or in Latin musculus psoas major, is part of the inner hip muscles.

It causes the internal and external rotation, lateral bending and flexing of the spine.

The Right Nutrition

Why is the right nutrition so important?

A healthy and balanced diet is of great importance for the perfect six pack. Every human being has muscles. The question is, how they are developed and how many layers of fat is on top of them.

Anyone thinking that he will get ripped abs just with working out alone is really mistaken. The key to a perfect six pack is the right diet, the workout for your muscles, and the heart- and circulatory exercise. One does not work without the other and does not produce the right results.

A balanced diet does not necessarily mean losing weight, but also building muscles, putting on weight. Without the proper nutrients you can't build muscles and will only add fat to your body.

What you need to pay attention to in your diet:
1.   Eat smaller meals

2.   5-6 meals throughout the say spread about 3 hours apart.

3.   Avoid binges by spacing the meals properly

4.   Fruit and vegetables are great to slow down your appetite.

5.   Drink a large glass of water before every meal

6.   Eat a lush and extensive breakfast

7.   Keep your dinner rather small and try to avoid carbs

8.   A big lunch will make you tired and cause problems to focus

    afterwards.

9.   Speed up your metabolism and burning fat with smaller meals

10. Every meal should contain proteins

11. Drink enough liquids, 2-4 liters; this will tone your muscles

12. Try to avoid eating in front of the TV or computer as you will eat more

13. Don't skip any meal as you will sabotage your balance

14. Healthy fats should be incorporated in your meals

15. Drink skim milk instead of full fat

16. Try to avoid fatty foods and eat more whole grain, vegetables and fruits.

Nutrients

Nutrients are essential organic or inorganic components. Nutrients are absorbed and processed through your metabolism.

They are divided into the following categories:

1. Vitamins
2. Minerals
3. Fat
4. Protein
5. Carbohydrates
6. Water

Vitamins

Vitamins are organic components which are important for the metabolism. Most of them can't be produced by your organism. They have to be added through nutrition. There are fat soluble and water soluble vitamins.

Vitamins have the task to regulate the recycling of carbohydrates, minerals, and proteins. They are also used to create energy, and are essential to build cells, bones, teeth, and blood cells, as well as strengthen the immune system. Vitamins can also be anti-oxidants.

An overview about vitamins will shed some light in the dark:

- VITAMIN A, also called Retinol, is part of the fat soluble vitamins. The daily requirement is between 0, 8 - 1 mg. You will find vitamin A in: liver, cod liver, fish, spinach, apricots, carrots, and honey dew melon, milk fat and as pro-vitamin in many plants. Vitamin A has an impact on eyesight, cell growth, and regeneration of the skin. Lack of vitamin A will lead to decreased visual acuity, night blindness, cornification of the visual cells, damage to skin and mucous membranes, susceptibility of the infectious system, and the stunt of growth in children. Overdosing on vitamin A during pregnancy can cause harm to the embryo and over many years it can lead to bone loss and osteoporosis.

- VITAMIN B1 also known was Thiamin is part of the water soluble vitamins. The daily requirements are 1.3 – 1.8 mg. Vitamins B1 is contained in yeast products, ham , brewer's yeast, whole grain bread, whole grain rice, honey, garlic, peas and meat. This vitamin is important for the nerves, the metabolism of carbs, thyroid function, the heart, and it is also a nutrient for the brain. Lack of vitamin B1 can lead to inflammation of the nerves, memory loss, depression, and heart insufficiency. Even more concentrated lack of vitamin B1 can cause Beriberi. Too much B1 has not been proven to cause any damage or side effects.

- VITAMIN B2, the so-called Riboflavin, belongs to the water soluble vitamins and the daily requirement is 1.8 – 1.0 mg. The following foods contain this vitamin: lean meats, milk, whole grain, cheese, eggs, spinach, cabbage, honey, fish, veal liver, and leafy greens. Vitamin B2 is very important for mother and child during pregnancy, enhances memory, important for concentration, helpful against strong migraines, blood formation in the skin forming tissue. Lack of vitamin B2 can cause Pellagra. As there are a variety of different and unspecific symptoms it is best to consult a physician if you think you are lacking B2. An overdose is not dangerous and there are no known side effects.

- VITAMIN B5 is also called pantothenic acid. The daily required doses is 8 -10 mg. Vitamin B5 is contained in whole grain products, eggs, veal liver, roasted peanuts, raw broccoli, meats (chicken and dark meats), peas, whole milk, and corn. Vitamin B5 strengthens the immune system, and promotes healing of wounds. It also acts as anti-stress factor, protects from x-rays, and is important for the transformation to the coenzyme A. Deficiency of vitamin B5 will cause problems with the healing of wounds and anemia. If Vitamin B5 is consumed in high doses over an extended period of time it can cause problems with digestion. .

- VITAMIN B6 is also known as Pyridoxine, belongs to the water soluble vitamins and the daily requirements is 1,6 – 2,1 mg. It is contained in liver, kiwi potatoes, meat, carrots, peas, fish, yeast, and oatmeal and rice meal. Vitamin B6 helps with the protein metabolism, prevents nerve damage, helps with pre-menstrual problems and bloating, infertility, prevents kidney stones, aids painful and stiff joints, and helps tearing. The lack of B6 leads to hypochromic anemia. Overdosing has no side effects on your body.

- VITAMIN B7is called Biotin and is part of the water soluble vitamins. The daily requirement is 0.25 mg. This vitamin is contained in cauliflower, liver (beef, veal, chicken, and lamb), leafy greens, porcini mushrooms, brewer's yeast, whole grain products, beef kidneys, soy beans, and button mushrooms. Vitamin B7 is important for skin, hair, nails, oil glands, aides the metabolism (forming of fatty acids and glucose).There is hardly ever a deficiency of vitamin B7. In the rare occasion it should happen you will experience loss of appetite, sickness, and scaly skin. In an extreme situation it can lead to loss of hair. Overdosing has no side effect.

- VITAMIN B9 is very well known as Folic Acid, a water soluble vitamin with a daily requirement of 0.16 to 0.40 mg. It is contained in the following foods: liver, pumpkin, wheat germ, Brussels sprouts, chick peas, spinach, green cabbage, asparagus, mandarins, white cabbage, leafy greens, yeast, eggs, salad, oranges and legumes. Folic acids are very important during pregnancy as it helps to prevent deformities of the unborn child. It is also important for the skin and muscle building. Lack of vitamin B9 can lead to pernicious anemia, change in mucous membranes, digestion problems, infertility, and problems with the unborn child during pregnancy. A dosage above 15 mg daily could lead to mood problems and trouble sleeping.

- VITAMIN B12 or Cobalamin   belongs to the water soluble vitamins and the daily requirement is 3µg. Cobalamin is contained in beef offal such as liver, kidney, and tongue, egg yolk, milk, herring, cheese, lean beef, and lupines. Vitamin B12 is important for the nerve functions, builds and regenerates red blood cells, increases appetite and is important for the building of protein based material. A deficiency will cause pernicious anemia and affects fertility. There are no known effects of overdosing \

- VITAMIN C or ascorbic acid is a water soluble acid. You should take 100mg every day. It is contained in rose hips, buckthorn, citrus fruits, kiwi, peppers, acerola cherries, kale , currants, tomatoes, sprouts, broccoli, strawberries, etc. Vitamin C almost has one of the most significant tasks in our body – maintaining a good immune system will prevent infections, is a radical scavenger, and has strengthening effect on the connective tissue. A deficiency is manifested by increased susceptibility to disease or scurvy. An overdose has no side effects.

- VITAMIN D also called Calciferol or Cholecalciferal is a fat soluble vitamin and the daily requirement is about 5 µg. This vitamin is produced by the body itself through UV-influence. Besides this you will find it in fish liver oil, beef and pig liver, tuna fish, sardines, herring, egg yolk, butter, and cheese. The most important task is to promote the absorption of calcium, as well as the regulation of the calcium metabolism and phosphate metabolism, besides this it strengthens the skeleton. Deficiencies can lead to rickets. A really high dose can even lead to death as the calcium is deposited in the body and will not be sufficiently excreted.

- VITAMIN E also called Tocopherol or Tocotrienol. It is part of the fat soluble vitamins and the daily requirement is about 10-15 mg. Vitamin E is contained in whole grain products, vegetable oils and nuts (peanuts, almonds, pecan nuts, hazelnuts). The function of vitamin E is cell regeneration, inhibition of inflammatory processes, wound healing, strengthening of the immune system, cardiovascular strengthening and is a radical scavenger. A deficiency is very rare; however, if it should occur, the nervous system, blood, muscles and vascular system will be affected. A really strong overdose can lead to stomach pain and diarrhea

- VITAMIN K also known as Phyllochinon, is a fat soluble vitamin of which the body requires 0,001 – 2 mg per day. You will find vitamin K in spinach, eggs, milk, potatoes, liver, lean meat, cabbages, broccoli, nettles, strawberries, tomatoes, and kale. It is effective against loos of calcium and aides the blood coagulation factors 2, 7, 9, and 10 A. Deficiency can lead to coagulation disorders and cerebral hemorrhage in newborns. An overdose of natural vitamin K will not harm the body, but artificial vitamin K can cause disorders of the blood coagulation. .

Minerals

Minerals are inorganic and organic substances of vegetable and animal origin. They are divided into volume elements and trace elements. As already identified by the name volume elements can be found more abundant in the body and trace elements, also called micro elements will be found in lesser quantities.

Volume elements are calcium, chlorine, cilium, magnesium, sodium, phosphor and sulfur.

Trace elements are chromium, iron, flour, iodine, cobalt, copper, manganese, molybdenum, nickel, selenium, vanadium, zinc and tin.

Below a brief overview about the most important functions of the individual minerals:
- Calcium is of essential importance for building bones and teeth, as well as the transmitting of nerve impulses.
- Chlorine helps building stomach acid and regulates hydrologic balance.
- Calium maintains the hyrdologic balance and regulates the heartbeat, as well as blood pressure, and aides the transmission of nerve impulses.

- Magnesium aides with the transmissions of the nerve impulses as well as muscle contraction. Bones and teeth contain magnesium.
- Sodium keeps the fluid balance in check as well as the nerve and muscle functions.
- Phosphor aides keeping bones and teeth healthy, and releases energy in cells.
- Sulfur is in all the cells as well as in protein substances.
- Chromium regulates the cholesterol and blood sugar levels.
- Iron is contained in hemoglobin and many enzymes.
- Fluor, is known by every child because of caries. It is necessary for the caries prophylaxis.
- Iodine is very important for the thyroid because it is a part of thyroxin (a thyroid hormone)
- Cobalt functions as enzyme activator and is part of vitamin B12.
- Copper helps bones and connective tissue to grow, and is needed to absorb iron.
- Manganese helps with the formation of bone tissue. It is contained in enzymes which are very important to transform energy.
- Molybdenum is involved in the production of DNS and RNS and is part of the enzymes.
- Nickel is also contained in DNA and RNA.
- Selenium protects cells from free radicals.

- Vanadium helps bones and teeth to grow.
- Zinc is found in enzymes and spurs regular growth, as well as influencing the immune system and fertility.
- The function of tin is not quite clear yet.

Fats

Fats are nutrients with the highest caloric value, approximately 39 kJ/g. They are of vegetative and animal origin and are divided into the following categories:

Saturated Fats – it is recommended that these fats are consumed in small quantities, as they are very quick to be noticeable on your hips, rips and in the loin area. Pockets of fat are created which are very difficult to get rid of. Saturated fats are most common to be found in meats and dairy products. However, you cannot completely skip these fats, as they also contain important nutrients. You can pay attention not to eat too much fatty meat and use lean meat and skim milk.

- Polyunsaturated fatty acids are among the recommended fats. They are subdivided into 2-fold, 3-fold, 4-fold, and 5-fold unsaturated fatty acids. The most commonly known polyunsaturated fatty acid is the Omega-3-fatty-acid, a 3-fold polyunsaturated fatty acid. It protects against cardiovascular disease and may help with weight control. This fat is most commonly found in fish, which also contains many valuable lean proteins for muscle building. Hence fish is twice as valuable and healthy for a great six pack

- Mono saturated fatty acids are most commonly found in vegetable oils (nuts, olives, avocados, pumpkin seeds, sunflower seeds, Safflower, linseed, hazelnut, canola, walnut). They lower cholesterol, promote the burning of fat, and prevent heart disease.

Protein

Proteins are also known as albumen. They are important nutrients for the entire body and its basic functions. Proteins carry out the task of building muscles, bones, organs, and connective tissue, support the digestive process, alert the body when nutrition should be used as energy or as fat deposits, provide part of the oxygen transport through the blood to various organs and muscles, and can also function as anti-body.

Protein can be of vegetable or animal origin. Animal proteins are very similar to human proteins. They are found in meat, fish, eggs, dairy products, legumes (beans, soy beans, peas, lentils…) and potatoes. The consumption of proteins enables the body to burn calories twice as fast as they are broken down into energy.

This in turn does not mean, if you only consume proteins your fat will melt completely. You still have to put your emphasis on a balanced nutrition; otherwise you will encounter other problems.

Carbohydrates

Carbohydrates are combined of carbon, hydrogen, and oxygen, and are produced by photosynthesis in plants. They are an important source of energy for the body as most of the cells use glucose as energy source.

Carbohydrates are also an energy reserve.

Carbohydrates are divided into simple sugar (Monosaccharide), double sugar (Disaccharide) and multiple sugars (Polysaccharide). Glucose –(fruits and vegetables), Fructose - (fruit and honey) and Galactose – (milk) are part of the simple sugar.

Beet sugar, cane sugar - sucrose (sugar beet, sugar cane, sugar, candy), milk sugar - lactose (milk, milk products), and malt sugar - maltose (barley, beer, malt extract) is one of the double sugar. Fall within the multiple sugar: starch (cereals, potatoes, and legumes), glycogen (liver, muscles) and cellulose (all plants).

Water

Water is a nutrient without which we could not survive. The human body consists of up to 70% water. If you drink too little water it can result in dehydration. A lack of fluid in the body is also manifested by dizziness, headache, muscle cramps, circulation problems and / or vomiting.

An excessive i.e. extremely high water intake can also lead to complaints about a so-called water intoxication. The daily recommended amount of water is between 1.5 to 4 liters. It all depends on the activities conducted and health.

The food groups

We divide our nutrition into groups to get a better overview and to be able to compose our diet plan much easier.

It is recommended that the main meals are comprised of three items from the food group and snacks should contain two items. This is also the foundation for a balanced nutrition.

Following a brief overview of the food groups:

- Leafy vegetables
- Legumes, beans
- Nuts
- Peanut butter
- Dairy products
- Eggs
- Oatmeal
- Whole grains
- Lean meats
- Olive oil
- Berries

Leafy vegetables

It is suggested to not to fry leafy greens or to prepare them with fatty cheeses because this will cause the most important vitamins and minerals will be lost. The most valuable leafy greens are spinach, broccoli, cabbage and Brussels sprout, yellow, green and orange vegetables (peppers, green beans, and asparagus).

These greens, most of all spinach, contain vitamin C, K and A, calcium, magnesium, and folic acids, beta carotene and roughage. These substances help to prevent cancer, being overweight, strokes, heart disease, and osteoporosis.

Legumes, beans
Bean dishes can replace meat once a week. In this group you will find: lentil, soy beans, chick peas, peas, kidney beans, butter beans, black and green beans.

This food group is rich in fiber, iron, folic acid, and protein. The group helps to build muscle, to burn fat, control digestion, and weight, as well is an excellent aid against heart disease, hypertension and colon cancer.

Nuts
This food group is very helpful for building muscles and as stomach filler, as well as aid against heart disease, regulates weight, and prevents cancer, wrinkles and hypertension.

Nuts come in a wide variety, such as: walnuts, peanuts, hazelnuts, pumpkin seeds, sunflower seeds, avocado, almonds, etc. They contain various amounts of protein, vitamin E, fiber, magnesium, phosphor, folic acids and mono saturated fatty acids. You should be more careful with roasted and salted nuts.

Peanut butter

Peanut butter is made from peanuts, just like the name suggests. It is rich in protein, vitamin E, niacin, mono saturated fatty acids and magnesium. Almond butter and cashew butter are very similar to peanut butter. They all prevent loss of muscle, wrinkles, being overweight and heart / circulation disease.

As this food group is also very rich in protein it helps building muscle and promotes burning fat. But you need to pay attention to the high fat and calorie content. Daily consumption should be limited to two or three tea spoons.

Dairy Products

Milk, yoghurt, cheese are dairy products. This food grou p is very attractive because it's high content of calcium, vitamin A, vitamin B12, riboflavin, cilium, and phosphor.

In general dairy products aid weight loss, strengthens the bones, prevents hypertension, cancer and osteoporosis as well as regulates weight.

Eggs

Proteins found in eggs are the best ones for the body. They promote muscle building the best. Eggs do not just contain protein, but also vitamin A and B12. This food group also regulates weight gain, du to high protein content.

Oatmeal

Breakfast cereal without sugar syrup, glucose syrup, and /or corn syrup is the best. Oatmeal contains complex long-chain fiber and carbohydrates. They are helpful against diabetes, heart disease, colon cancer, and control the blood sugar level as well as cholesterol and weight.

Whole Grain Bread

This group contains all the whole grain products which are made of real whole grain and where vitamins, minerals and fibers have already been reduced due to industrial processing.

Whole grain products are very filling because of the complex carbohydrates they contain. In addition to this they are also full of vitamin E, B2, B1, B6, protein, fiber, and minerals (magnesium, iron, cilium, calcium, and zinc). This mix of nutrients prevents storing of fat ni the body, hypertension, being overweight, heart disease, and cancer.

Lean Meat

Those kinds of meat contain protein, zinc, iron, vitamin B12, phosphor, and cilium. Additionally beef contains creatine; fish is rich in Omega-3-fatty acids, and the vitamin B6 is found in chicken and fish.

This food group is ideal for strengthening of the immune system, building muscles, and to fight being overweight. When consuming beef you should rather chose a piece of the topside, rump steak, or beef filet because of the high proportion of saturated fatty acids.

Turkey breast and mussels also belong to this food group. Fish has the highest Omega-3- fatty acid content and is best suited to lower the lepton level in our blood. This in turn leads to better burning of fat, i.e., metabolism. Besides this it is excellent to prevent prostate cancer.

Olive Oil

Walnut oil, pumpkin seed oil, hemp oil, sunflower seed oil, linseed oil, hazelnut oil, canola oil, sesame oil, peanut oil, and safflower oil also belong to this group. Those oils have a high content of mono unsaturated fatty acids and vitamin E. Olive oil, as well as the other oils, help fighting against hypertension, heart disease, being overweight and cancer.

Berry Fruit

Apples and grapefruit are close relatives of berries. They contain vitamin C, fiber, anti-oxidants, and ketamine (not all of them). Berries have a protective effect against heart disease, and are helpful for better vision, balance, coordination and short term memory, as well as protect against binging and cancer.

Tips how to consume fewer calories

and additional nutritional hints.

A balanced diet is the non plus ultra. We will provide you with some helpful tips how you can consume fewer calories and increase burning body fat. New knowledge pops up everywhere, or even some of your grandmother's old home remedies are helpful tips for your diet. But now down to business.

1.   Tip – Lemon juice

Taking about 3 TL lemon juice before a meal can lower the blood sugar reaction from the meal about 10%. It is important to use freshly pressed lemon juice. Lowering the blood sugar lever will extend your body's fat burning mode. This will also prevent cravings.

2.   Tip - Cinnamon

Cinnamon as well helps to lower the blood sugar reaction, in some cases up to 29% after a consumed meal. Following some variations of cinnamon: Vietnamese cinnamon has the strongest reaction, in second place you find cassia cinnamon, and in third place Ceylon cinnamon. Cinnamon is often used as spice and is ideal for yoghurt and oatmeal. It is also very harmonious with apples and almond butter. There is a level for cinnamon consumption which should not be exceeded and is approx. 4 grams.

3.   Tip – Beef or bison meat

There is a huge difference between grass-fed animals, and animals fed with corn and soy beans. The first have the healthier meat as the others were exposed to an altered feeding pattern, which led to a higher content of Omega-6-fatty acids and not enough Omega-3-fatty acids. .

In addition those meats contain three times less vitamin E than grass-fed animals. This meat does not only more vitamin E but also a healthy fat called CLA (conjugated linoleic acid). CLA helps the body for burn fat and builds lean muscles. The proteins have a high quality and spur burning fat. You can't find any disadvantages in this meat. .

4.   Tip – Avocados

They are full of healthy fats, as well as minerals, vitamins and anti-oxidants. The Mexican dip, Guacamole, is made of mashed avocado, garlic, onions, tomatoes, and other ingredients to your taste. It tastes delicious on bread with scrambled eggs, or even with salad. This dip is nutritious and tasty.

5.   Tip – Whole eggs

They are the biggest source of protein and also contain calcium, lutein, iron, zinc, phosphor, folic acid, vitamin B6, B12, A, D, E, K, and B1, as well as essential fatty acids. You should always pay attention to buy farm fresh eggs, where the chicken are not laying their eggs in farming batteries, as the quality will not be the same.

6.   Tip – Nuts

They are fatty nutrients, however, they contain healhty fat. Besides this they are rich with vitamins, minerals, fiber, protein and anti-oxidants. Nuts are perfect for cravings. They control appetite and blood sugar levels, which in turn leads to more efficient burning of fat, and lower caloric intake. Untreated nuts are better than salted and roasted ones.

Well known nut products are peanut butter, walnuts, hazelnuts and pecan nut butter. There are peanuts, walnuts, hazelnuts, almonds, cashews, pecans, and many other varieties.

7.   Tip – Berries

Strawberries, raspberries, blackberries, blueberries, and other berries are full of minerals and different vitamins and also contain a variety of anti-oxidants. They are excellent for digesting carbohydrates because of their fiber.

Berries keep your body lean. They are an excellent snack together with yoghurt or cottage cheese, or just in muesli. But they still taste best fresh and on their own.

8.   Tip – Mustard family vegetables
A lot of people won't know about this name, but they will know broccoli, Brussels sprouts, kale, cauliflower, or cabbage. These vegetables are great for fighting stomach fat. Even if not so popular, it has a great effect in fighting estrogen combinations which can wreck the body's equilibrium.

9.   Tip – 20 minutes before your meal
It is recommended to eat a handful of nuts about 20 minutes before any meal. Your brain will register a decrease in appetite because you have already taken in a healthy portion of calories with good fatty acids. Any kind of nut is fine. With this simple trick you will eat smaller portions and lose more body fat.

10. Tipp – The scents of food

Peppermint and vanilla are great to reduce your appetite. Simple put a couple drops of peppermint on a napkin and sniff a couple times, or put up some vanilla scented candles around you. You can lose about 230g of fat per week.

11. Tip – Smaller plates and smaller silverware

According to a study people eat more from larger plates and bigger silverware than smaller ones. Your eyes will see a full plate, which will also be registered by your brain and send the signal to eat everything.

If your plate is smaller it is full as well, but there is less on the plate an in the end the brain will get a signal when you finish everything on the plate – my plate is empty, I am full. Don't wait, get a smaller plate and smaller silverware. And – no second helping!

12. Tip – Eating speed

Our brain only registers after approximately 20 minutes that we are full and we should use this knowledge. You start out with a normal eating speed and then slow down to half the speed. This will result in eating a smaller portion, but you will still feel full.

13.   Tip – Out of sight - out of mind

Try to avoid having junk food in your house in order to eat healthy foods. Don't put chocolate on the table as this will result in eating six times as much as putting it further away. Am besten kein Junk Food im Haus haben, denn dann essen Sie gesunde Nahrungsmittel. Schokolade nicht direkt auf den Tisch legen, denn so isst man circa sechsmal mehr als wenn sie weiter weg liegt.

14.   Tip – No distraction

You will eat about 15% less, if you eat in peace and quiet and without any distraction (TV, computer...). Of course you will be full and satisfied, maybe even more so, because you were able to enjoy your meal without any distraction.

Diet Plan and Recipes

A smart diet plan consists of 5-6 meals per day. One day a week can be figured in as a day with guilty pleasures. The special thing about it is that you will not eat according to any plan. Following a couple recipes for your meals:

You are able to combine them and built your own diet plan. It is really of advantage to set up a 14 day diet plan. Your nutrition should be diversified and contain a variety of foods.

Recipes for breakfast

1.   Ham and mushroom omelet with an orange on the side
Ingredients: 3 slices of Serrano ham, 3.5 oz. mushrooms and 5 egg whites, 1orange
Preparation: Cut the ingredients in small pieces and fry them briefly in olive oil, add the 5 egg whites, season according to taste.

2.   Apple-rice with a slice of whole grain bread and cottage cheese

Ingredients: 1.7 oz. rice, 1 apple, 1 tsp. spoon fresh lemon juice, cinnamon, slice of whole grain bread and cottage cheese.

Preparation: Cook the rice in 200 ml water, shred the apple and mix with the lemon juice. Mix the shredded apple with the rice and season with cinnamon and honey.

3.   Tuna fish omelet with non-fat plain yoghurt

Ingredients: 1 egg, 4 egg whites, some lemon juice and water, 1 can of tuna fish, 1 tbsp. whole grain flower and 1 tbsp. small oats, non-fat yoghurt

Preparation: Form a dough with egg, egg whites, water, lemon juice flower and oats. Fry on both sides and fill with tuna fish.

4.   Yoghurt bomb with a small apple

Ingredients: 7 oz. Greek yoghurt, 3 tsp. spoon oats, 1 tbsp. raisins, 1 tsp. diet jelly and a small apple

Preparation: Mix all ingredients and ready us your breakfast!

5.   Cottage cheese with berries and a kiwi

Ingredients: 5.5 oz. cottage cheese, 3.5 oz. berries (strawberries, blackberries raspberries etc.), 20 peanuts or almonds and 1 kiwi

Preparation: Mix all the ingredients – ready you are!

6.   Whole grain bread with an apricot on the side

Ingredients: 2 slices whole grain bread, 1 egg, 2 walnuts, low fat cottage cheese, 4 leafs of Romaine lettuce and an apricot

Preparation: Spread the cottage cheese on the bread; in the meantime boil the egg. Slice the egg and put it on the bread, top with salad and walnuts. Eat together with the apricot.

7.   Peach yoghurt with pistachios on the side half a tomato and some parmesan cheese.

Ingredients: 1 peach, 2 tsp. wheat germ, 3.5 oz. low fat plain yoghurt, 1 teaspoon pistachios

Preparation: Mix the yoghurt with the pistachios and the wheat germ. You can also mix in the peach, or eat it on the side.

8.   Yoghurt peanut butter with 15 hazelnuts on the side.

Ingredients: 7 oz. nonfat plain yoghurt , 1 small banana, 1 table spoon peanut butter (natural and low sugar), a pinch of cinnamon, 15 hazel nuts

Preparation: Cut the banana in pieces and mix it with yoghurt and peanut butter, season with cinnamon.

9.   Salsa-spinach-egg with 1 orange on the side

Ingredients: 4 egg whites, 4.5 oz. spinach (fresh or frozen), 3 tbsp. natural salsa, season to your liking and one orange on the side.

Preparation: Fry the egg whites with the salsa, heat up the spinach in the meantime, and serve everything on one plate.

10.   Tuna fish spread with one orange on the side

Ingredients: 1 can of tuna (without oil), 2.5 oz. cottage cheese, 1 slice of whole grain bread, 3 tsp. chives, capers, 1 orange

Preparation: Mix all ingredients except the orange and the slice of bread. Spread the mixture on the bread.

11.   Whole grain toast with one kiwi on the side

Ingredients: 2 eggs, 1 slice of whole grain bread , 1 tbsp. low fat mayonnaise, 1 tsp. mustard, 2 leafs Romaine lettuce, seasoning (water cress or chives and pepper) and 1 kiwi

Preparation: hard boil the egg, mix with mayonnaise, mustard, chives and other seasonings, spread onto the bread and garnish

12.   Fruit yoghurt

Ingredients: 1 natural yoghurt, 1 half a banana, 1 small apple, 2 tbsp. oats, 2 tsp. mixed nuts, pinch of cinnamon

Preparation: cut the fruit into small pieces and mix with the other ingredients.

13.   Egg vegetable salad with natural yoghurt on the side

Ingredients: 2 eggs, 3.5 oz. broccoli, 2.5 oz. canned corn, 1 small carrot, ¼ onion, spices, 2 tbsp. olive oil, 1 natural yoghurt

Preparation: mix all the ingredients together, except the yoghurt.

14.   Salsa-pepper omelet and half an apple on the side.

Ingredients: 1 egg, 3 egg whites, ¼ peppers (red or green), ¼ onions, 2 tsp. low sugar salsa, 1 slice of pumpernickel bread and ½ apple

Preparation: Mix the egg with the salsa, cut onion and pepper and fry lightly, mix the egg together with the onion and pepper to form an omelet. Once ready put it on the pumpernickel bread.

15.   Grits with milk and two table spoons of mixed nuts

Ingredients: 200 ml low fat milk, 0.7 oz. soft wheat grits, 1 small apple, pinch off cinnamon, 2 tbsp. mixed nuts.

Preparation: cook the grits in the milk, cut the apple in pieces and heat it in the microwave, pour the grits over the apple and sprinkle with cinnamon.

16. Crisp bread strawberries and one natural yoghurt on the side

Ingredients: 4 slices crisp bread, 2 tbsp. natural peanut butter, 5-7 strawberries and 1 natural yoghurt.

Preparation: Spread the peanut butter on the crisp breat and put the sliced strawberries on top.

17. Egg-vegetable omelet with a side of natural yoghurt

Ingredients: 1 egg, 3 egg whites, 125 g frozen mixed vegetables,

1 natural yoghurt

Preparation: Stir fry the vegetables lightly, add egg and egg whites while mixing everything. Season to taste.

18. Cottage cheese - yoghurt with 1 breakfast egg

Ingredients: 3.5 oz. cottage cheese, 3.5 oz. plain yoghurt, 1 kiwi and one breakfast egg

Preparation: Mix all the ingredients except the egg – enjoy!

19. Greek Yoghurt with berries and crisp bread with cottage cheese.

Ingredients: 3.5 oz. plain yoghurt, 2.5 oz. Greek yoghurt, 2 oz. mixed berries, 5-7 Almonds, 1 tsp. Cinnamon or diet jam , 1 crisp bread (Wasa), and cottage cheese

Preparation: Mix all ingredients except crisp bread and cottage cheese – enjoy!

20. Cornflakes with milk and an orange

Ingredients: 4-5 tbsp. sugar free cornflakes, 125ml milk (0,5% fat), 1 tbsp. protein powder, one orange

Preparation: Mix all ingredients except the orange.

21. Greek yoghurt with fruit

Ingredients: 4.5 oz. plain Greek yoghurt , ½ apple ,5 strawberries, 2 tsp. chopped walnuts, 4 tbsp. oats, 1 tsp. honey

Preparation: Cut fruit into small pieces, mix yoghurt and honey adding the fruit and other ingredients.

22. Whole grain bread with egg and 1 kiwi

Ingredients: 1 slice whole grain bread, 3 egg whites, 1 tbsp. diet mayonnaise, 2 leaves Romaine salad, 1 slice low fat cheese and 1 kiwi

Preparation: Spread the mayonnaise on the bread, put fried egg whites, salad and cheese on top.

23. Yoghurt with protein powder and one small banana

Ingredients: 4.5 oz. plain yoghurt, 1 tbsp. protein powder, 2 tbsp. sunflower seeds, a small banana

Preparation: mix all ingredients, if you like you can also slice the banana and add it.

24. Egg whites, Pumpernickel bread and plain

Ingredients: 4 egg whites, 1 slice pumpernickel bread, 1 tsp. natural peanut butter, 2 leaves Romaine salad , seasoning , 1 plain yoghurt

Preparation: put the peanut butter and salad on top of the pumpernickel bread and tip with the fried egg whites.

25. Whole grain bread, turkey breast, plain yoghurt and walnuts

Ingredients: 2 slices whole grain bread, 2 slices low fat turkey breast, 4 small radishes, cottage cheese, 1 plain yoghurt, 1 walnut

Preparation: Spread the cottage cheese on to the whole grain bread top with turkey breast and radishes.

26. Romaine salad with egg and 1 kiwi

Ingredients: 4 egg whites, 2 tbsp. cottage cheese, 4 large leaves Romaine salad, 2 tsp. Salsa, 1 Kiwi

Preparation: Fry the egg whites, add salsa and cottage cheese, spread the mixture onto the Romaine salad leaves.

27.   Greek yoghurt with nuts and an apple
Ingredients: 5.5 oz. Greek yoghurt, 2 tbsp. hazelnuts, 2 tbsp. almonds, 1 EL diet jam, 1 apple
Preparation: mix all the ingredients except the apple and enjoy!

28.   Peanut butter crisp bread with banana
Ingredients: 1 plain yoghurt, 1-2 tbsp. peanut butter, 1 small tomato, 3 slices crisp bread (Wasa), 1 banana
Preparation: Slice the tomato, mix peanut butter with the yoghurt and spread onto the crisp bread. Put the sliced tomatoes on top of the bread

29.   Cottage Cheese with Pumpernickel and 1 apple
Ingredients: 4.5 oz. cottage cheese, 2 slices of pumpernickel bread, 2 leaves Romaine salad, 1 egg, 1 apple
Preparation: hard boil the egg, spread the cottage cheese on the bread and top with salad and sliced egg.

30.   Artichoke salad with plain yoghurt

Ingredients: 3.5 oz. artichoke hearts, ¼ red pepper, 1 can tuna fish, parsley or oregano, pepper, garlic, 1 plain yoghurt

Preparation: cut artichokes and peppers into small pieces and mix with the tuna, season to your liking.

31.   Egg spread with 1 kiwi

Ingredients: 3.0 oz. cottage cheese, 4 egg whites, 1 tsp. mustard, 1.5 oz. diced ham, fresh herbs, 1 slice pumpernickel, 1 kiwi

Preparation: fry the egg whites. Then mix all ingredients except the pumpernickel and kiwi. Spread the mix onto the pumpernickel and garnish with herbs.

32.   Turkey Breast sandwich and 1 pear

Ingredients: 2 slices whole grain bread, 1 tomato, 2 slices turkey breast, low fat parmesan, 2 tsp. olive oil , 1 pear

Preparation: Sprinkle olive oil onto the bread. Top with turkey breast and tomato, and sprinkle parmesan on top. Briefly heat up in the micro wave to melt the cheese.

33.   Greek yoghurt with granola and 3-5 strawberries

Ingredients: 5.5 oz. Greek yoghurt, 2 tbsp. Granola, 2-3 walnuts, 1 tsp. raisins, 3-5 strawberries

Preparation: mix all the ingredients, if you like you can also add sliced strawberries.

34.   Weight Gainer Shake
Ingredients: 5.5 oz. oats, 3.5 oz. Greek yoghurt, 300ml milk, 1-2 tbsp. honey, 1 banana
Preparation: mix all the ingredients in a blender

35.   Eggs with cheese or turkey
Ingredients: 2 eggs, 6 egg whites, 2-3 slices whole grain bread, low fat cheese or turkey breast
Preparation: Mix the eggs and egg whites and fry in a pan. Put the cheese slices or turkey breast on top of the bread and top with the eggs,

36.   Oat waffles and an apple
Ingredients: 7 tbsp. oats, 4-5 eggs, 1 handful raisins, 2 tbsp. sunflower seeds, one apple
Preparation: Mix all ingredients very well and fry in pan or griddle

37.   Scrambled eggs with bacon
Ingredients: 4-6 eggs, bacon, 2-3 slices of whole grain bread
Preparation: mix eggs and scramble in a pan, brown bacon in a separate pan and top eggs with bacon.

The first snack between meals

Plain yoghurt

Ingredients: 1 plain yoghurt, 2 tsp. oats, 1 tsp. diet jam

Preparation: mix everything together and enjoy!

2.   Peach with almonds

Ingredients: 1 peach, 7 almonds, 1 tsp. raisins

Preparation: cut the peach into small pieces mix with the other ingredients and enjoy.

3.   Rice cake with boiled ham

Ingredients: 2 rice cakes, 3 tsp. cottage cheese, 2 slices lean ham

Preparation: Spread the cottage cheese on to the rice cakes and top with boiled ham

4.   Mango with peanut butter

Ingredients: ¼ mango, 3 tsp. peanut butter

Preparation: Slice the mango and dip them into the peanut butter.

5.   Rice cake with peanut butter

Ingredients: 1 rice cake, 1 tsp. peanut butter, 1 tsp. cream cheese, 2 radishes

Preparation: Spear the peanut butter and cream cheese on the rice cake and top with radishes.

6.   One orange

7.   Crisp bread (Wasa) with herbs
Ingredients: 1 crisp bread, 2 tsp. cottage cheese, fresh herbs, 1 radish, 4 slices fresh cucumber
Preparation: Spread the cottage cheese on to the crisp bread and top with herbs, radish, and cucumber.

8.   One apple

9.   Plain yoghurt with nuts
Ingredients: 1 plain yoghurt, 8-10 diced nuts, 1 tbsp. diet jam
Preparation: mix all the ingredients and enjoy.

10.   Small fruit salad
Ingredients: ½ banana, ½ apple, 2 tsp. raisins, 8-10 almonds
Preparation: Slice fruit and almonds in pieces and mix together.

11.   Cashews with Greek yoghurt

Ingredients: 3.5 oz. low fat Greek yoghurt, 2 tsp. cashew nuts, 1 tsp. diet jam

Preparation: chop nuts into small pieces and mix with the other ingredients.

12.   Peanut butter shake

Ingredients: 1 tsp. peanut butter, 1 plain yoghurt, 2 tsp. oats

Preparation: Mix all ingredients in a blender, if you like add some crushed ice.

13.   Rice cake with cream cheese

Ingredients: 1 rice cake, 2 tsp. cream cheese, 1 slice turkey breast

Preparation: top the rice cake with all the ingredients.

14.   Apple with cottage cheese

Ingredients: ½ apple, 2 tbsp. cottage cheese

Preparation: slice apple in small pieces and mix with the cottage cheese.

15.   Oats with Greek yoghurt

Ingredients: 3.0 oz. Greek yoghurt, 2 tsp. oats, 1 tsp. diet jam

Preparation: Mix all the ingredients and enjoy.

16.   One banana

17.   Kiwi almond butter
Ingredients: 1kiwi, 2 tsp. sugar free almond butter
Preparation: Slice the kiwi and spread the almond butter on top of it.

18.   Rice cakes with Serrano ham
Ingredients: 2 rice cakes, 3 tsp. cream cheese, 2 slices Serrano ham, 2 leaves Romaine salad
Preparation: Spread cream cheese on the rice cakes and top with ham and salad

19.   Crisp bread with lox
Ingredients: 2 slices crisp bread, 1 slice lox, 2 tsp. cream cheese, 2 leaves Romaine salad
Preparation: Spread the cream cheese on the crisp bread and top with lox

20.   Plain yoghurt with almonds
Ingredients: 1 plain yoghurt, 6-8 almonds
Preparation: chop the almonds and mix them into the yoghurt

21.   Apple & Pear with Mozzarella

Ingredients: ½ apple, ½ pear, 50g mozzarella, 5-7 almonds,

1 tsp. olive oil

Preparation: Cut all the ingredients in small pieces and mix together.

22.   Cornflakes with milk

Ingredients: 125ml fat free milk, 4 tbsp. sugar free cornflakes, 2 tbsp. oats, 2 tsp. raisins

Preparation: mix all the ingredients with the milk.

23.   Yoghurt with sunflower seeds

Ingredients: 1 plain yoghurt, 2 tsp. sunflower seeds, 1 tbsp. protein powder

Preparation: mix all ingredients.

24.   Crisp bread with egg

Ingredients: 1 crisp bread, 1 egg, 1 tsp. cream cheese, 2 radishes, fresh herbs

Preparation: hard boil the egg and top the crisp bread with all the ingredients.

25.   Yoghurt with cinnamon

Ingredients: 1 plain yoghurt, 3 tbsp. mixed nuts, 1 tsp. cinnamon

Preparation: just mix all the ingredients

26.   Apple with cheese

Ingredients: ½ apple, 1.5 oz, cucumber, 1 low fat sliced cheese, 1 tbsp. chopped pine nuts , 1 tsp. olive oil

Preparation: Cut apple, cucumber and cheese into small pieces and mix with the remaining ingredients.

Lunch recipes

1.   Whole grain roll with lox

Ingredients: 1 whole grain roll, 2.5 oz. smoked lox , 3.0 oz. cream cheese, fresh herbs, 2 leaves Romaine salad, ½ tomato, seasoning

Preparation: mix fresh herbs, lox, and cream cheese in a blender and spread onto the rolls top with salad and tomato.

Whole grain roll with egg and tomato

Ingredients: 1 whole grain roll, 4 egg whites, 2 tsp. tomato paste, 2 tsp. parmesan cheese, 1 tbsp. salsa (sugar free)

Preparation: Use the egg whites for scrambled eggs and add the tomato paste. Put the salsa on the roll, top it with the scrambled egg and parmesan cheese. Slide it in the oven to melt the cheese.   Parmesan, jetzt noch kurz in den Ofen schieben, damit der Käse zergeht und fertig

Turkey breast the quick way

Ingredients: 3 oz. turkey breast filet, 1 baked potato, 3.5 oz. green beans, 1.7 oz. carrots, 2.5 oz. broccoli

Preparation: cook the baked potato in the oven. Fry the remaining ingredients in a pan with some olive oil and season to taste. Plate together with the potato

Whole grain ham sandwich

Ingredients: 1 whole grain roll, 2 slices Serrano ham, ½ tomato, 2 tsp. diet mayonnaise, 1 slice sandwich cheese

Preparation: use all the ingredients to make a delicious sandwich.

Chicken breast with rice

Ingredients: 3.5 oz. chicken breast , 3 oz. brown rice, 1.5 oz. cucumber, 2 leaves iceberg lettuce, 1.5 oz. carrots (canned or frozen), seasoning

Preparation: cook the rice. Fry the chicken breast on both sides and put it in the oven for 15 minutes. Prepare the carrots in a roux. Put the carrots and cucumbers on the salad and season according to your taste.

6.   Chicken breast filet

Ingredients: 3.5 oz. boneless chicken breast, 1 potato, 5 Asparagus spears, 3 tsp. parmesan cheese, 1 tsp. diet mayonnaise, olive oil and seasoning according to taste.

Preparation: Season the potato and chicken breast, broil in the oven for 25 minutes. Sprinkle parmesan and heat it up briefly in the microwave. Plate everything together.

7.   Turkey breast and pineapple salad

Ingredients: 4.5 oz. turkey breast, 1.7 oz. iceberg lettuce, 1.7 oz. pineapple chunks, 1.7 oz. canned corn, 1 tbsp. tomato paste, 1 tbsp. diet mayonnaise, seasoning.

Preparation: cut the turkey breast in small pieces, season them and briefly fry them in a pan. Add the remaining ingredients except the iceberg lettuce and let simmer until cooked through. Put everything on top of the lettuce.

8.   Fried herring with Greek yoghurt

Ingredients: 4.5 oz. fried herring (marinated in oil and vinegar), 1 baked potato, 4 tbsp. low fat Greek yoghurt, 1-2 tsp. linseed oil, parsley, chives, seasoning

Preparation: bake the potato in the oven, plate everything together, put the Greek yoghurt and linseed oil on top of the potato, season with herbs and garnish with the herring.

9.   Vegetable salad with turkey breast

Ingredients: 4 slices turkey breast , 1 small tomato, 2 tbsp. canned corn, 4 leaves Romaine salad, 3 tbsp. mixed nuts, 2 tsp. raisins, 2-3 tsp. Sesame oil

Preparation: chop the nuts and cut all the other ingredients in small pieces. Mix everything together, add oil, and season to your taste.

10.   Tuna fish hamburger

Ingredients: 1 can of tuna, 2 egg whites, 2-3 tbsp. oats, 1 tsp. chopped onions, some oatmeal, 1 tsp. salsa

Preparation: Mix all the ingredients together, except the salsa, and form hamburger patties, fry them and use the salsa as sauce.

11.   Turkey strips with rice

Ingredients: 3.5 oz. turkey, 3.5 oz. brown rice, 1.2 oz. sliced mushrooms, 1.2 oz. corn, 1.2 oz. peas (canned or frozen), 1 tbsp. walnut oil, seasoning

Preparation: cook the rice, cut the turkey in strips, season and brown. Add the remaining ingredients and cook another 10 minutes.

Plate everything together with the rice.

12.   Omelet with turkey

Ingredients: 1 egg, 2 egg whites, 2 two slices turkey breast , 4 tbsp. cooked chick peas, 3 tsp. cream cheese, 2 leaves iceberg lettuce,

¼ onion

Preparation: spread the cream cheese on top of the lettuce, combine the remaining ingredients and make an omelet.

13. Whole grain roll with scrambled eggs

Ingredients: 1 whole grain roll, 4 egg whites, 2 tsp. diet mayonnaise, 6 cucumber slices, 1 slice of sandwich cheese

Preparation: make scrambled eggs from the egg whites, spread the cream cheese on the roll, put the scrambled egg on the roll and garnish with the cucumber.

14. Whole grain roll with tuna

Ingredients: 1 whole grain roll, 1 can tuna fish, 1 egg white, 2 tsp. cream cheese, 3 oz. mixed vegetables, seasoning.

Preparation: Spread the cream cheese on the whole grain roll, fry the tuna together with the egg whites and put them on the roll. Saute the vegetables lightly and plate together with the roll

15. Shrimps with delicious sauce

Ingredients: 8 large cooked shrimp, 1 baked potato, 3 oz. cream cheese, 1/4 red pepper, 1/4 onion , seasoning

Preparation: Bake the potato in the oven, the shrimp are already cooked. Put the remaining ingredients in a blender and mix until they are creamy, serve together with the shrimp as delicious sauce.

16.   Tuna fish ratatouille

Ingredients: 1 can tuna fish (in water) , ½ onion, 1 bell pepper, ¼ zucchini, 1 small tomato, rosemary, basil , garlic, seasoning

Preparation: Cut all the ingredients in small pieces, finely chop the onion, and mix everything together. Put everything on a baking sheet and bake in the oven for approximately 20 minutes.

17.   Baked pork tenderloin

Ingredients: 3.5 oz. pork tenderloin , 2 slices turkey breast , 3 oz. button mushrooms, 1 small baked potato, 1 large leaf iceberg lettuce , seasoning and perhaps some cream cheese as sauce.

Preparation: Brown the tenderloin and wrap with the slices of turkey breast, then continue to fry together with the button mushrooms. Put everything together in the oven on a baking sheet for approximately 25 minutes.

Bake the potato as well. Serve everything together on the leaf of iceberg lettuce.

18.   Quick filet of trout

Ingredients: 6.5 oz. filet of trout, ½ tomato, 2.5 oz button mushrooms, ¼ zucchini, celery, 1 tsp. walnut oil , seasoning

Preparation: Cut all ingredients in small pieces, except the fish. Cover a baking sheet with tinfoil and baste it with the oil. Put the filet on top of the cut vegetables and close the tinfoil. Let it steam for 20 minutes in the oven

19.   Rolled pickled herring - the simple way

Ingredients: 1 baked potato, 4.5 oz. rolled pickled herring (in brine) , 2 tsp. parmesan cheese, 2 leaves Iceberg lettuce, seasoning

Preparation: Oven-bake the potato and cut into pieces, top with shredded parmesan cheese and plate on top of the lettuce with the herring on the side.

20.   Beef filet with mushrooms

Ingredients: 6 oz. lean beef or veal, 3.5 oz. oyster mushrooms , 1 tbsp. parmesan cheese, ½ onion or shallot , 1 tbsp. cream cheese , seasoning

Preparation: Cut all ingredients into small pieces, sauté lightly in a pan except the parmesan. Put the everything together in a casserole dish , sprinkle parmesan over it and back for 20 minutes. The cream cheese can be used as sauce.

21.   Prawns in a pan

Ingredients: 5.5 oz. cooked prawns without shell, 1 orange, 1 leaks stalk, 1 oz soybean sprouts, 1 tbsp. sweet chili sauce , 1-2 tbsp. sesame oil , Muscat, seasoning

Preparation: Cut the orange and soybean sprouts into small pieces, slice leak into rings. Steam leak and soybean sprouts in the heated sesame oil for about 5 minutes, add prawns an orange sauté another 5 minutes. Season with Muscat and sweet chili sauce.

22.   Salmon with tomatoes

Ingredients: 5.5 oz. salmon filet, 1 small tomato, ¼ onion, 1.7 oz. cream cheese, basil, rosemary, seasoning

Preparation: Use the cream cheese as dip. Thinly slice the tomato and dice the onion. Put both on a baking sheet with tin foil. Then put the salmon on top. Close the tinfoil and bake about 20 minutes in the oven.

23.   Turkey breast with rice

Ingredients: 3.5 oz. Turkey breast, 3.5 oz. brown rice, 3.5 oz. broccoli, ½ tomato, 2 tsp. diet mayonnaise, seasoning

Preparation: Season the broccoli and wrap it into tin foil, put in the oven for about 20 minutes. Cook the rice, season the turkey brreast and sautee in olive oil . Plate everything together and use the tomato to garnish, diet mayonnaise as sauce.

24. Whole grain burger

Ingredients: 1 Whole grain roll, 2 Slices turkey breast, 2 tsp. Cream cheese, ½ tomato, ½ pickle, 1 tsp. mustard, parsley or chives, seasoning

Preparation: Mash the turkey slices together with the cream cheese and mustard in a blender, spread onto the whole grain roll, garnish with slices tomatoes and pickle.

25. Pork tenderloin with broccoli

Ingredients: 3 oz. Pork tenderloin, 4.5 oz. broccoli, 2 tsp. parmesan cheese, 1 slice whole grain bread, 2 tsp. cream cheese with chives, seasoning

Preparation: Season the pork tenderloin and sauté in a pan, put shredded parmesan cheese on top of it. Plate all together.

26. Chicken Nuggets

Ingredients: 5.5 oz. Boneless chicken breast, 2 egg whites, 2 tsp. salsa, ½ cup flower, 1 cup cornflakes smashed into crumbles, cream cheese, seasoning

Preparation: Cream cheese will be used as sauce/dip. Cut the chicken breast in medium sized pieces and dip into the flower. Mix the egg whites with salsa and dip the chicken pieces in it. At last roll the chicken pieces in the cornflakes crumbles. Put into pre-heated oven for about 10 minutes or until golden brown.

27.   Cod filet with vegetables

Ingredients: 7 oz. cod filet, 5.5 oz. mixed vegetables, seasoning

Preparation: the vegetables will be sautéed in a pan. Bake the seasoned fish covered in tinfoil for approximately 15 minutes in the oven. Plate everything together.

28.   Turkey breast with rice – 2nd receipe

Ingredients: 5.5 oz. Turkey breast, 5.5 oz. Brown rice, 1 small tomato, seasoning

Preparation: while cooking the rice cut the turkey breast into pieces and sauté in oil. Slice the tomato as garnish and plate everything together.

29.   Tuna fish with potato

Ingredients: 1 can tuna fish (in water), 1 baked potato, 1.2 oz. chick peas, 2 leaves iceberg lettuce, seasoning

Preparation: drain the tuna and sauté in a pan, mix with the chick peas. Bake the potato and place on the lettuce, top with the tuna and chick peas.

30.   Vegetable egg sandwich

Ingredients: 5 Egg whites, 2.5 oz. diced red pepper, 1 oz. finely chopped onion, 1 slice pumpernickel, 1 tsp. salsa, 1.7 oz. cucumber, seasoning

Preparation: briefly sauté the onion and pepper and mix with egg whites and salsa. Put the entire mixture on top of the pumpernickel and garnish with cucumber.

Snack after lunch

1.   Protein shake 1

Ingredients: 3 tsp. protein powder , 1 tsp. Stevia, 2 tsp. Greek yoghurt, water, crushed ice (optional)

Preparation: Put everything in a blender and mix.

2.   Protein shake 2

Ingredients: 3 tsp. protein powder, 1 tsp. plain yoghurt, 2 tsp. cottage cheese, water

Preparation: mix everything in a blender, crushed ice optional

3.   Protein shake 3

Ingredients: 2 tsp. protein powder, 1 tsp. Stevia, ½ banana, water

Preparation: mix everything in a blender

4.   Protein shake 4

Ingredients: 2 tbsp. protein powder, 1 tsp. Stevia, 2.5 oz. mixed berries, water

Preparation: mix in a blender and enjoy

5.   Protein shake 5

Ingredients: 3 tsp. protein powder, 1 tsp. natural honey, water

Preparation: mix everything in a blender

6.   Protein shake 6

Ingredients: 2 tsp. protein powder, 1 tsp. dextrose, ½ peach, water

Preparation: mix in a blender

7.   Protein shake 7

Ingredients: 3 tsp. protein powder, 1 tsp. Stevia, water

Preparation: mix in a blender, crushed ice optional

8.   Protein shake 8

Ingredients: 2 tsp. protein powder, 1 tsp. honey, 2 tsp. oats, 2-3 strawberries, water

Preparation: mix everything in a blender, crushed ice optional

9.   Protein shake 9

Ingredients: 2 tsp. protein powder, 1 tsp. dextrose, 1 tsp. peanut butter, water

Preparation: mix everything together in a blender

10.   Protein shake 10

Ingredients: 2 tsp. protein powder, 1 tsp. honey, 2.5 oz. mixed berries, water

Preparation: mix everything in a blender, crushed ice optional

11.   Protein shake 11

Ingredients: 3 tsp. protein powder, 1 tsp. dextrose, water

Preparation: mix in a blender, crushed ice optional

12.   Protein shake 12

Ingredients: 2tsp. protein powder, 1 tsp. honey, 2.5 oz. pineapple, water

Preparation: mix together in a blender

13.   Protein shake 13

Ingredients: 2 tsp. protein powder, 1 tsp. dextrose, 3 tbsp mixed berries 1 tsp. peanut butter, Water

Preparation: Mix everything together in a blender

14.   Protein shake 14

Ingredients: 2 tsp. protein powder, 1 tsp. Honey, 100ml pineapple juice, water as necessary

Preparation: mix everything in a blender

15.   Protein shake 15

Ingredients: 2 tsp. protein powder, 2 EL low fat yoghurt, ¼ mango, 1 tsp. stevia, water

Preparation: mix everything in a blender

16.   Protein shake 16

Ingredients: 2 tsp. Protein powder, 3 tbsp. mixed berries, 1 tsp. dextrose, water

Preparation: mix everything in a blender

17.   Protein shake 17

Ingredients: 2 tsp. protein powder, ½ banana, 1 tsp. dextrose, water

Preparation: mix everything in a blender

18.   Protein shake 18

Ingredients: 2tsp. Protein powder, ¼ mango, 1 tsp. Stevia, water

Preparation: mix everything in a blender

Diner recipes

Fish filet with vegetables

Ingredients: 4.5 oz. fish filet according to choice, 1 small bell pepper, ½ onion, 1 small tomato, 3 oz. broccoli, and seasoning

Preparation: Brush a baking dish with oil. Cut the vegetables into small cubes. Put the fish in the baking dish and cover with the vegetables, brush lightly with oil and season according to taste. Bake for 20 minutes in the oven.

Chicken with watercress

Ingredients: 3 oz. Boneless chicken breast , ¼ cucumber, ½ chives or onion, 3 tbsp. water cress, 4 leaves lettuce, 1 tsp. raisins, 1 tsp. pine nuts , 1 tsp. sunflower seeds, 2 tsp. olive oil, seasoning

Preparation: wrap the chicken breast in tinfoil and braise it in the oven, season according to taste. Dice the cucumber and mix it with the sunflower seeds, pine nuts, and raisins. Plate everything together.

Egg and vegetable omelet

Ingredients: 1 egg, 4 egg whites, 4.5 oz. mixed vegetables, 2 tbsp. cream cheese, seasoning, olive oil
Preparation: Mix all the ingredients and put it in a pan to make an omelet.

Salad with shrimp

Ingredients: 3.5 oz. Cottage cheese, 8-10 cooked shrimps, ½ tomato, ½ orange, 6 leaves romaine salad, 1 tsp. soy sauce, 2 tsp. sesame oil, seasoning
Preparation: cut the tomato, salad and orange in small pieces, mix everything together and season with soy sauce, sesame oil. Top with cottage cheese and shrimps.

Tuna fish tortillas

Ingredients: 1 can tuna fish (in water), 3 egg whites, 2 oz. bell pepper, ¼ onion, 1 tomato, finely chopped parsley, seasoning

Preparation: finely dice the onion and bell pepper and sauté, add tuna fish and parsley and the egg whites. Season according to your taste. Bake everything togehter and garnish with seasoned tomatoes.

Cottage cheese with pineapple

Ingredients: 4.5 oz. Cottage cheese, 2.5 oz. Pineapple, 2 tbsp. Mixes nuts, 2 slices turkey breast, fresh herbs, seasoning

Preparation: dice the turkey breast and mix with the other ingredients and enjoy.

Baked cod filet

Ingredients: 1 cod filet, ¼ bell pepper, ¼ onion, 2 oz. broccoli, ½ cup milk, 1.7 oz. cream cheese, fresh herbs and seasoning acc. to taste.

Preparation: prepare the sauce from cream cheese, fresh chopped herbs, and milk. Dice onion and bell pepper and put on tin foil basted with oil. Put the cod filet on top. Close the tinfoil and bake for approximately 20 minutes.

Tuna fish with mixed vegetables

Ingredients: 1 can tuna fish, 3.5 oz., mixed vegetables, 2 tbsp. salsa, seasoning

Preparation: Mix all ingredients and sauté in a pan. Season according to taste.

Shrimps with vegetables

Ingredients: 8-10 cooked shrimps, 1.7 oz. peas, 1.7 oz. carrots, 1.7 oz. corn, 3 tbsp. cottage cheese, 1 tsp. salsa, seasoning

Preparation: mix cottage cheese and salsa and serve as dip. Briefly sauté the shrimp and vegetables and plate everything together.

10.   Vegetable rice salad

Ingredients: 1.7 oz. brown rice, 2 slices boiled ham, 3 oz. mixed vegetables, ½ tomato, ¼ onion , 3 tsp. cottage cheese, seasoning

Preparation: Cook the rice and dice the other ingredients and sauté.

11.   Turkey meatballs

Ingredients: 4 oz. ground turkey, 2 egg whites, ½ onion , ½ whole grain roll, 1 tsp. mustard, 1 tsp. tomato paste, seasoning

Preparation: chop the onion in small pieces, soak the roll in water and press water out of it. Mix all the ingredients, season, and form little balls, which will be fried in the pan.

12.   Fish salad with beans

Ingredients: 3.5 oz. Fish filet (according to choice), 1.7 oz. cooked garbanzo beans, ¼ onion, or chives, ½ tomato, ½ bell pepper, 1 tbsp. cream cheese, seasoning

Preparation: season the fish filet and sauté in a pan. Cut the vegetables in small pieces and sauté in a pan. Add cream cheese and plate everything together.

13.   Chicken Sandwich

Ingredients: 3 oz. boneless chicken breast, 2 slices of whole grain bread, ¼ onion, 1.7 oz. button mushrooms, 2 leaves Romaine salad, 1 slice of cheese, 2 tsp. diet mayonnaise, ½ tsp. mustard, seasoning

Preparation: toast the whole grain bread. Cut the onion and button mushrooms and sauté, mix mustard and diet mayonnaise and spread on the toasted bread. Fry the chicken breast and put on top of the toast.

14.   Turkey and ham salad

Ingredients: 2 slices turkey breast, 2 slices ham, 2 slices cheese, 1.7 oz. zucchini, ¼ onion , ½ apple, seasoning

Preparation: dice all the ingredients and mix together, add olive oil and season to taste.

15.   Chicken strips with bell peppers

Ingredients: 3.5 oz. boneless chicken breast, ½ red bell pepper, ¼ green bell pepper, 1 small tomato, ¼ onion, ½ cup chicken stock, some white wine, 1 splash lemon juice, seasoning

Preparation: cut bell peppers, onion, and chicken breast in strips and sauté the chicken breast in the pan after you season it. Cook the bell pepper and onion, add the remaining ingredients. At last add the chicken breast strips and let cook briefly.

16.   Baked white fish

Ingredients: 4.5 oz. White fish, 1.7 oz. brown rice, 2.5 oz. broccoli, 2 slices of cheese, 1 tsp. walnut oil, seasoning

Preparation: season the white fish and broccoli and bake 20 minutes in the oven. In the meantime cook the rice and sprinkle with walnut oil. Shortly before the fish comes out of the oven put the cheese slices on and let them melt on top of the fish. Serve on a plate with the rice.

17.   Tomatoes with meat filling

Ingredients: 2 tomatoes, 3.5 oz. cottage cheese, 2 oz. leaks, 4 slices turkey breast, fresh herbs, seasoning and 1 tbsp. walnut oil

Preparation: dice all the ingredients except of the tomatoes and mix them together. Season to taste, hollow out the tomatoes and fill with the mixture, bake for 25 minutes in the oven.

18.   Turkey filet with rice

Ingredients: 3 oz. turkey breast filet, 2.5 oz. brown rice, 2 leaves iceberg lettuce, 1.5 oz. canned corn, seasoning
Preparation: season the turkey breast filet, wrap in tinfoil and bake in the oven. Cook rice and corn. Plate everything on top of the salad.

19.   Toast with turkey breast
Ingredients: 2 slices whole grain bread, 4 slices turkey breast, 2.0 oz. button mushrooms, 2 slices Gouda cheese, ¼ onion, 2 tbsp. diet mayonnaise, seasoning
Preparation: slice button mushrooms and onion. Spread the mayonnaise on the bread and top with all the remaining ingredients. Put the bread in the oven and let the cheese melt on top of it.

20.   Salmon vegetable salad
Ingredients: 3.5 oz. smoked lox, 1 small tomato, ½ bell pepper, ¼ onion, 3 walnuts (chopped), 2 tsp. olive oil, and seasoning
Preparation: dice all the ingredients and mix together, season according to taste.

21.   Crisp bread with cottage cheese
Ingredients: 2 slices of crisp bread, 3 oz. cottage cheese, 2 leaves Romaine salad, ½ tomato, seasoning

Preparation: Spread the cottage cheese on the crisp bread, and put the remaining ingredients on top of it, season to taste.

22.   Turkey strips with mushrooms
Ingredients: 3.5 oz. turkey breast, 1.5 oz. button mushrooms (can, 80ml vegetable stock, 40ml milk, olive oil, red wine, seasoning
Preparation: cut the turkey breast and mushrooms in small pieces and sauté in a pan; add the vegetable stock and some red wine. Let simmer for a couple minutes, add seasoning and mix in the milk.

23.   Turkey & pineapple with cottage cheese
Ingredients: 4.5 oz. cottage cheese, 2.5 oz. pineapple chunks, 2 tbsp. mixed nuts, 2 slices turkey breast, fresh herbs, seasoning
Preparation: cut the turkey breast and pineapple chunks and mix with the other ingredients.

24.   Turkey hamburger with peppers
Ingredients: 4 oz. ground turkey, ½ bell pepper, seasoning, 3.5 oz. celery, 1 oz. peas
Preparation: roast the bell pepper, then cut in fine pieces together with the celery. Mix all the ingrdients and season. Form a patty and fry.

25.   Jacket potato with curd cheese

Ingredients: 2 small boild potatoes, 4.5 oz. cream cheese with chives, 3 tbsp. Mixed nuts, 2 oz. mountain cheese, 1-2 tsp. linseed oil, seasoning

Preparation: Mix all ingredients except potatoes. Plate and put the potatoes on the side

26.   Chicken breast with vegetables

Ingredients: 3.5 oz. boneless chicken breast, 3.5 oz. mixed vegetables, seasoning, 1 tbsp. diet mayonnaise

Preparation: season the chicken breast and sauté, add the mixed vegetables and let simmer about 10 minutes. Use the diet mayonnaise as twister.

27.   Fried squid rings with rice

Ingredients: 3.5 oz. calamari, 2.5 oz. brown rice, 4 leaves Romaine salad, 1 tsp. salsa, 2 tsp. diet mayonnaise, seasoning

Preparation: mix salsa and diet mayonnaise for the sauce, cook the rice, fry the calamari, plate everything together on top of the salad.

28.   Shrimps with vegetables

Ingredients: 6-8 large cooked shrimp, 2.5 oz. broccoli 1/2 onion, 1.7 oz carrots, 1/2 bell pepper, 2 tsp. salsa, olive oil, and seasoning

Preparation: dice all the vegetables very fine and put them in the oven together with the shrimp, before coat everything with olive oil, cook about 15 - 20 minutes. You can either mix the salsa in the dish or pour over top.

29.   Salmon with potatoes

Ingredients: 5.5 oz. salmon filet, 1 small potato, 2 oz. broccoli, 2 tbsp. cream cheese, fresh herbs, seasoning

Preparation: finely chop the herbs and add them to the cream cheese, prepare as dip. Season the salmon, potato and broccoli and bake in the oven for about 20 minutes.

30.   Cod filet with lentil

Ingredients: 1 cod filet, 3.5 oz. lentil, 1.7 oz. cream cheese, ½ dried chili pepper, some garlic, 2 tbsp. sesame oil, seasoning

Preparation: cook and season the lentils, mix with chili, garlic and cheese. Season the cod filet and saute . Plate everything together.

31.   Beef strips with broccoli

Ingredients: 3 oz. lean beef, 1 shallot, 2 tbsp. cream cheese, 1 tsp. salsa, 3.5 oz. broccoli, and seasoning

Preparation: mix salsa and cream cheese for a dip. Cook the broccoli wrapped in tinfoil in the oven. Cut the beef in strips; slice the onion and sauté with oil.

32. Haddock balls

Ingredients: 4.5 oz. haddock filet, 3.5 oz. cream cheese, 2 egg whites, ½ onion, fresh herbs, some wheat flower, a dash of white wine, seasoning.

Preparation: Put all the ingredients except the white wine and flower in a blender, mix until you have a smooth mass. Roll into meatball size, coat with flower. Boil water and add a splash of white wine, cook the balls for approximately 10 minutes.

33. Crabmeat with avocados

Ingredients: 2 small avocados, 11 oz. crab meat, 2 tbsp. lemon juice, 1.7 oz. cucumber, 1/2 chili pepper, 2 tbsp. olive oil , seasoning

Preparation: dice avocados, chili and cucumber, sauté together with the crab meat in a pan. Mix lemon juice, oil and sesoning as dressing.

Snack after diner

Cottage cheese with herbs

Ingredients: 2.5 oz. cottage cheese, 6 almonds, 2 tsp. parsley or chives, seasoning

Preparation: finely chop almonds and herbs and mix with the cottage cheese.

Eggplant with cream cheese

Ingredients: 2 small eggplants, 2 oz. cream cheese, seasoning

Preparation: spread the cream cheese on top of the eggplants and season to taste.

Plain yoghurt with protein powder

Ingredients: 2.5 oz. plain yoghurt, 2 tsp. protein powder, ½ banana

Preparation: cut the banana in small pieces and mix with the remaining ingredients.

Avocado with peanut butter

Ingredients: 2 avocado slices about 1 inch thick, 1 tbsp. peanut butter.

Preparation: spread the peanut butter on top of the avocado slices.

Cottage cheese with blueberries

Ingredients: 2.5 oz. cottage cheese, 2 tbsp. blueberries

Preparation: just mix both ingredients together.

Apple with sunflower seeds

Ingredients: ½ apple, 2 tsp. sunflower seeds

Preparation: cut the apple in small pieces and mix with the sunflower seeds.

Yoghurt with peach

Ingredients: 2.5 oz. plain yoghurt, 1 tsp. protein powder, 1/2 peach

Preparation: cut the peach in small pieces and mix with the other ingredients.

Olives with dip

Ingredients: 8-10 olives, 1 tsp. salsa, 1 tsp. cream cheese

Preparation: mix cream cheese and salsa and serve as dip with the olives.

9.   Yoghurt with almonds

Ingredients: 2.5 oz. plain yoghurt, 5-7 almonds, 3 tbsp. raspberries

Preparation: chop the almonds and mix with the remaining ingredients

10.   Orange with peanut butter

Ingredients: 1 small orange, 2 tsp. peanut butter

Preparation: break or cut the orange in pieces and spread the peanut butter on top of it.

11.   Cottage cheese with apple
Ingredients: 2.5 oz. cottage cheese, ½ apple
Preparation: cut the apple in small pieces and mix with it with the cottage cheese.

12.   Greek yoghurt with hazelnuts
Ingredients: 2.5 oz. low fat Greek yoghurt, 2 tsp. protein powder, 2 tbsp. hazel nuts
Preparation: chop the hazelnuts and mix with the other ingredients.

13.   Peanut butter shake
Ingredients: 100ml low fat milk, 2 tsp. peanut butter
Preparation: put everything in the blender and mix - enjoy your shake!

14.   Cottage cheese with mango
Ingredients: ¼ mango, 2 tsp. cottage cheese.
Preparation: cut the mango in small pieces and mix with the cottage cheese.

15.   Yoghurt with pineapple

Ingredients: 2.5 oz. plain yoghurt, 1.7 oz. pineapple, 1 tsp. protein powder

Preparation: cut the pineapple in small pieces and mix withthe remaining ingredients.

16.   Cottage cheese with walnuts

Ingredients: 2 oz. cottage cheese, 4 chopped walnuts, 1 tbsp. diet jam Preparation: mix all the ingredients together

17.   Rice cake with ham

Ingredients: 1 rice cake, 2 tsp. cream cheese, 1.7 oz. smoked ham, 1 leaf Romaine salad

Preparation: spread the cheese on top of the rice cake and put the ham on top of it.

18.   Apple with mixed nuts

Ingredients: ½ apple, 2 tsp. mixed chopped nuts, 1 tsp. sunflower oil

Preparation: cut the apple in small pieces and mix everything together.

19.   Greek yoghurt with strawberries

Ingredients: 2.5 oz. low fat Greek yoghurt, 3-5 strawberries

Preparation: cut the strawberries into pieces and with the yoghurt.

20. Yoghurt with sunflower seeds

Ingredients: 2 oz. plain yoghurt, 2 tsp. sunflower

Preparation: mix all the ingredients together.

21. Cucumber with cream cheese

Ingredients: 4 cucumber slices about 1 inch thick, 2 tsp. cream cheese, cayenne pepper

Preparation: spread the cheese on the cucumber slices and season with cayenne pepper.

22. Greek yoghurt with peach

Ingredients: 2 oz. low fat Greek yoghurt, ½ peach, 2 walnuts

Preparation: chop the walnuts and cut peaches in small pieces and mix into the yoghurt

23. Yoghurt with pistacchios

Ingredients: 2.5 oz. plain yoghurt, 2 tsp. pistachios

Preparation: finely chop the pistachios and mix into the yoghurt

24.   Peach with peanut butter

Ingredients: 1 small peach, 2 tsp. peanut butter

Preparation: either slice the peach and spread the peanut butter on the slices, or dice the peach and mix with peanut butter

25.   Orange with almonds

Ingredients: ½ orange, 3 tsp. almonds

Preparation: finely chop the almonds, cut orange into small pieces and mix together

26.   Kiwi with peanut butter

Ingredients: 2 tsp. peanut butter, 1 kiwi

Preparation: slice the kiwi and spread the peanut butter on it , or dice the kiwi and mix with the peanut butter.

All the recipes are suggestions. In your diet plane you can change diner recipes to lunch or vice versa or even combine different ingredient. The most important factor is that you will have a well-balanced diet plan.

You can see the big variety to choose from, now it is your turn to be smart in trying everything and enjoy eating! Everyone carries a six pack, just like we mentioned before, but a lot of times it is hidden under a small layer of fat.

You can't just work off this layer. By eating smart you can have it melt away. Working out is the dot on the "i" and will polish the diamond in the rough.

Workout Plan

General workout plan.

Every six pack work out needs to include working out your entire body, cardiovascular training, some strength training, and the targeted six pack work out.

Each of the training / work out should consist of the following three phases:
- warm up
- main training session
- cooling down or stretching- and relaxing exercise

In order to really build great muscles everyone has to rest. The muscles will not grow during the work out, but in the phases of resting.

To alternate your exercises is just as important as working out on a regular basis. It does not matter whether you work out at home or in the fitness studio, with or without equipment.

Make sure to avoid abrupt movements, the speed and repetitions are not really very important. It is much more important to exercise slowly and do it right. This will stimulate the muscles and will let them grow.

After time exercises will seem too easy for you, even if you are following a professional plan and you should use more weights. This will make sure that your exercises will be more difficult.

The work out plan for beginners contains about 2-3 sets for each exercise, intermediate 2-4 sets and advanced will do 5-7 sets. Each set consists of 10-15 repetitions of the same exercise. The breaks in between will also get shorts the longer you are working out. Beginners will take a break of 1 ½ to 2 minutes, professionals will only take a 45-60 second break.

Maybe this sounds a little funny, but to really get the perfect six pack you don't have to work out your abs that much. It is much better to work out your entire body and do a couple targeted abdominal exercises.

You need your abdominal muscles to walk, sit, and stand. This means that you will use this muscle group with everything else you do, like doing squats, lifting, walking, push-ups etc. Not in vain you will hear inhale, exhale, and tighten your stomach in order to do an exercise the right way.

Cardiovascular Training

The cardiovascular training is a very important part of burning fat and stimulates the body to burn off calories. But there are some rules that everyone should pay attention and stick to in order to get the best benefit.

Just like the name says, this work out is for the cardiovascular system. It is supposed to strengthen the heart and activate the metabolism. This will encourage the fat burning process.

Some of the most important rules in an overview:
-	Do not go above 65% of the maximum stress factor.
-	While you are exercising you should still be able to chat.
-	Work out regularly.
-	Adjust intensity and duration of your work out to your body.

Walking, swimming, jogging, bicycling etc. are considered cardiovascular workout. It is important to pay attention to the warm up, core exercise and cool down.

Following some interesting ways to exercise indoors or outdoors, with and without equipment:

1.   You can power walk without any major expenditure, all you need is being in a good mood and passion. It is suitable for everyone , it's easy on the joints and still uses about 660 muscles in your body. Power walking is not normal walking or jogging, it is something in between. You should start with normal walking and increase the speed gradually, then slowdown in the end. After the walking you need to stretch your arms and legs.

2.   You can inline skate with rollerblades (inline skates). It is an activity which is done outdoors most of the time.

3.   Jogging is considered to be endurance training. As with everything else you should pay attention and not overwork yourself. You should still be able to chat while you are jogging. Always stretch after you are jogging. Breathing right is very important.

4.   Swimming is very demanding and healthy for your entire body. Everyone has their very own style. Again you need to pay attention to breathe right and not overwork yourself. Overworking yourself does not get

you any better results, quite the opposite; it is not recommended at all.

5.   Almost everyone knows bicycling. It may be a sport, a past time, or jst a way to move around. Being part of cardiovascular workout the three known phases are absolutely necessary.

6.   Rowing is a sport which is done with a certain kind of boat. There are different boat classes. There are two different techniques, sculling or oar rowing.

7.   Squash – tennis –badminton – soccer – basketball – table tennis, these are all sport which are also played professionally. With all of them you are not playing alone, but with another player or in a team.

8.   Aerobic is a mixture between gymnastics and dance. The exercise, which is called choreography, is done with music.

9.   Spinning – most of the time this is done in a fitness studio. Of course you can also buy a spinning bike for your home gym. Most of them are equipped pulse- and frequency meter, as well as with programs for cardiovascular training.

10.   Steppers – can replace power walking and have built in programs for cardiovascular exercise, which makes things a lot easier. However, this does not replace stretching after exercising.

11.   Treadmill – can replace walking or jogging outdoors because you can do it indoors or in the gym. Most of the modern treadmills come with programmed exercises.

12.   Ergometer – replaces rowing on water and you can do it at the gym when the weather is bad. But like with everything else you need to pay attention to warm up and cool down.

You should start out exercising about 20 minutes and slowly increase the time.

Full body training

Full body training means to exercise your entire body. All your muscle groups are stimulated and build up.Ganzkörpertraining bedeutet den ganzen Körper zu trainieren.

The body is segmented in the following muscle groups:

- Arms
- Shoulders
- Stomach
- Back
- Legs

All those muscle groups are again separated in a finer classification. This will be explained in detail discussing the individual groups.

Arms

Biceps

1.   Arm curl variation 1 – Stand with your feet at shoulder width apart. Take a barbell or two smaller dumbbells. Your arms are beside the body, without being stretched all the way. Now they are drawn to the shoulder and return to the starting position.

2.   Arm curl variation 2 – Stand with your feet shoulder width apart. Stretch your arms horizontally away from your body with your palms facing up. You can use dumbbells and curl your arms in a 90 degree angle towards your head. Then return into the starting position.

3.   Hammer Curl – Stand with your feet shoulder width apart. Extend your arms alongside your body almost all the way. Take two dumbbells. Your palms are facing your body. Curl your forearms up to a 90 degree angle. Then return to the starting position.

4.   Arm curl variation 3 – Elbows braced on a bench. Palms facing down. Take a dumbbell in each hand. Pull your lower arms up to your face up to 90 a degree angle.

Triceps

1.   Arm stretching behind the body. Stand shoulder width apart. Take two dumbbells and stretch your arms behind your back. Pull your lower arms up to a 90 degree angle, and then stretch them out again.

2.   Arm stretching above your head – Stand shoulder width apart.

Stretch your arms above your head with a dumbbell between them. Bend your arms backwards and pull them up again.

3.   Arm stretching on an incline bench – Sit down on the incline bench. Take a dumbbell in each hand and bend your forearms towards your back. Then stretch the arms out above your head.

4.　　Arm stretching obviated – support yourself by putting one arm and one knee on a bench, keep the other leg on the floor. Take a dumbbell and keep your hand parallel to your body. Now move your forearm to the front in an angle no more than 90 degrees.

Dips

1. Variation 1 – Take two benches. Support yourself with your arms stretched out, put your feet on the other one. Lower your body to the ground and lift it up again into the starting position.

2. Push-ups – place your arms shoulder width apart at chest height.　Your legs are straight and only your toes are on the ground. The arms are stretched out. Your entire body is in the air except your toes and your palms. Lower your body towards the ground and remain straight like a board. Lift it back into the starting position.

3. Push-ups with one hand – Everything is the same as above. Except that you do the pushups with one hand.

Wrists

1. Variation 1 – stand with your feet shoulder width apart. Take two dumbbells . Your arms are stretched out in front of your body. Palms are facing your body. Pull the dumbbells up from your wrists and bring them back to the starting position.

2. Variation 2 – The same as above except that the palms are facing away from your body.

Shoulders

Front shoulder muscles

1. Front lifts variation 1 – Stand shoulder width apart. Stretch your arms besides your body. Pull the stretched arms up horizontally. Then bring them back into the starting position.

2. Front lifts variation 2 – Everything is the same as above, except that you are alternating working with your arms.

3. Front lifts variation 3 – Everything is the same as in variation 1, except that you take a bigger dumbbell and use both hands. Pull both hands at the same time horizontally in front of your body and bring them back into the starting position.

Medium shoulder muscles

1. Lateral raise – Stand shoulder width apart. Both hands stretched out beside your body. Take two dumbbells. Pull your arms horizontally and pull them up a little further, always keeping your arms stretched out completely. Now bring your arms back into the starting position.

2. Military press variation 1 – Stand shoulder width apart. Take one dumbbell and stretch your arms vertically above your head. Now pull them down. Your upper arm will be in a horizontal 90 degree angle to your lower arm. Then lift them back up. Your palms are facing to the front the entire time.

3. Shoulder press variation 2 – Everything is the same as in variation 1 , except that your palms will point towards your ears.

4. Shoulder press variation 3 – Everything is the same as in variation 1, except that you are sitting down.

1. Shoulder press variation 4 – Everything is the same as in variation 2, except that you are sitting down.

Back shoulder muscles

1. Variation 1 – Stand shoulder width apart, slightly bend your knees. Schulterbreiter stehen, leicht in die Knie

gehen. Bend your upper body horizontally to the front. Take two dumbbells in your stretched out arms. Now pull your arms up horizontally. Return to the starting position

2. Reverse Butterfly – This exercise is done sitting on a bench. Grip the handles with both hands and pull your arms to the front.

Back

Lower back muscles

1. Eagle's flight – lay on your stomach, legs stretches out. Arms stretched out in front of your head. Lift up your upper body and pull your stretched arms to the side. Return to the starting position.

2. Eagle's flight variation 2 – everything is the same as in variation 1 , except that the arms are pulled all the way down to your buttocks and return to the starting position.

3. Upper body lift variation 1 – Lay on an incline bench. Put your arms behind your head. Bend your upper body down, pull it back up and lower it again. Then return to the starting position.

4. Upper body lift variation 2 – stand shoulder width apart. You're your upper body parallel to the ground. Your arms are stretched towards the ground. Take a dumbbell in each hand. Pull your body up while keeping your arms stretched out. Lower your body to the starting position

Middle back muscles

1. Pull ups with a wide overhand grip – use a pull up bar to pull yourself up and lower yourself again.

2. Pull ups with a narrow overhand grip – do this exercise on a pull up bar as well.

3. Rowing – you will find different equipment for this exercise at the gym.

4. Lats – stand shoulder width apart. Arms stretched out in front of your body with your palms facing your body. Take two dumbbells and pull your arms up, but no more than in a horizontal position. Lower them to the starting position.

Upper back muscles

1. Variation 1 – stand shoulder width apart. Position your arms stretched out behind your back with a dumbbell in

each hand. Your palms are facing outwards. Pull your shoulders up and lower them again.

2. Variation 2 – stand shoulder width apart. Stretch your arms in front of your body, your palms are facing towards your body. With a dumbbell in each hand pull your shoulders up and lower them again.

3. Rowing while standing up – stand shoulder width apart. Arms are stretched out in front of your body. Your palms are facing your body. Lift your elbows as far as possible. Your hands with the dumbbells remain in front of your body at chest height. Bring your arms to the starting position.

Legs

Upper leg muscles

1. Leg stretching on a machine – Sit on the bench and stretch the legs, then return to the sitting position.

2. Squats – stand shoulder width apart. Put your hands behind your head. Go into your knees and come back up.

3. Squats variation 2 – everything is the same as in variation, except you are using a long bar at the same time.

4. Squats variation 2 – stnad a little wider than shoulder width. Stretch your arms away from your body in a horizontal position with a dumbbell in each hand. Go down into your knees and bring your arms together. When getting back up also bring your arms back into the starting position.

Calves

1.   Heel lift option 1 – stand shoulder width apart. Hands beside your body. Lift up your heels and stand on your tiptoes. Lower your heels to the starting position.

2.   Heel lift option 2 – everything is the same as in option 1, except that you will lift one foot off the ground and do the exercise standing on one leg only.

3.   Heel lift option 3 – everything is the same as in option 1 , except using your arms dumbbells. .

Upper abdominal muscles

Below we are explaining a variety of exercises, with and without equipment. You can do them either at home or at the gym.

1.   Crunch – keep your legs angled on the ground – this exercise is easy on the back. Lie on the ground and place your hands on your temple while your feet are placed on the ground and your legs at an angle. Pull your upper body towards your knees. This exercise is slow and controlled . If you have reached your highest point halt for a couple seconds before you lower yourself down again.

2.   Crunch – with your legs lifted up – lie on the floor with your legs lifted up at a 90 degree angle. Palms on your temples again. Chin to your chest while your head remains lifted up with every variation of the crunch. Pull your upper body up towards you knees again . This exercise is also slow and controlled. At the highest tension point exhale and remain in this position briefly before returning to the starting position.

3.   Crunch – Put your feet on an elevated platform – in the gym you will have a special bench for this exercise, at home you may use a chair. Put your feet on the chair with your calves lying on the chair. This exercise is the same as all the other crunches. Lift your upper body, remain in the position and then go back to the starting position.

4.   Crunch – incline bench - lie down on the incline bench and put your palms on your temples. Pull your body up towards your feet for a few inches and remain in this tightened position briefly before returning to the starting position.

5.   Crunch – variation 1 for your upper abs – put your legs shoulder width apart and slightly bend forward while bending your back like a cat. This exercise is slow and controlled. Keep your head straight in the starting position and pull your chin to your chest during the exercise.

6.   Crunch – variation 2 for your upper abs – get on your knees and pull your upper body forward while you tighten your stomach muscles. Slowly return to the starting position.

7.   Crunch – lower abs – get on your knees, and bend your body toward the ground, tighten your stomach muscles. Each of those exercises should be slow and controlled.

8.   Lower abs variation 1 – get on your knees and sit down keeping your buttocks slightly above the calves. Your feet are at a 90 degree angle and your body is

almost parallel to the ground. Now lower your body towards the ground slightly further than in a horizontal position. This exercise is slow and controlled.

9.   Situp – on the ground – Lie on the floor and bend your legs, cross your hands on your chest or put your palms on your tamples. Pull your upper body up with your head towards your knees. The difference between crunch and sit up is a smaller movement. During a sit up your body is pulled up further than during a crunch. The crunch is easier on your back then the sit up. But the sit up has a lot more effect on your abs.

10.   Sit up – on the floor with weights – the entire exercise is the same as above, but you will use a weight on your chest.

11.   Sit up – incline bench – position yourself on the incline bench. Cross your arms on your chest or put your palms on your temples. Pull your upper body up very slowly and lower it down again.

12.   Sit up – incline bench variation 2 – everything like above, except you are using a weight on your chest to make this exercise a little more difficult.

13.   Sit up – with your feet elevated – you can use a chair at home, or appropriate equipment at the gym – put your hands in the same position as described above. Pull your upper body towards your knees. Remain in this position briefly and go back to your starting position. As always exhale at the point of greatest tension.

14.   Upper abs variation 3 – stand shoulder width apart. Bend down your entire upper body towards the ground while keeping your back straight. Keep it at a 45 degree angle. Return into the starting position.

Lower abdominal muscles exercises

For the lower abdominal muscles you will find a variety of exercises. Of course there are also a lot of variations.

1. Leg lift – ly flat on the ground with your legs stretched. Arms beside your body and slightly lift your legs off the ground. Then lift your legs all the way up in the air with your feet parallel to the ground. Lower your legs locking them in a position where they are about two inches off the ground. This exercise is also slow and very

controlled. Inhale when you lift your legs, exhale when you lower them.

2. Crunch with one leg at an angle – Position yourself lying on the ground. Put your feet against a wall at a 45 degree angle. Stretch your arms out facing away from your body. Straighten one leg and pull it towards your upper body, while lifting your arms off the ground. . Put your arms down and your foot back on the wall. Repeat the same exercise with the other leg.

3. Crunch with your legs bend - position yourself on the ground with your feet at a 45 degree angle off the ground and stretched out. You're your arms up and keep them parallel to the ground beside your body. Pull up your upper body and your angled legs at the same time. The basic motion is similar to rowing. Stretch your legs again and lower your body to the ground. Your arms will remain off the ground at all times.

4. Hip lift – lay on the ground with your arms stretched out beside your body lifting your legs straight up and keeping your soles parallel to the ceiling. Lift up your hips and lower them down again. You can put your hands under your back to make this exercise a little easier.

5. Jackknife exercise – lay flat on the ground, stretch your arms out behind your head, stretch your legs. Your arms and legs won't touch the ground when you start this exercise. Keeping your back straight you wull start to lift up your upper body with stretched arms while also lifting your legs up at the same time. Just like trying to touch the tip of your toes with your fingertips. Return to your starting position. This exercise is slow and very controlled as well as being highly effective.

6. Jackknife exercise for beginners – lay on the ground, stretch your arms out behind your head and leave your legs at an angle with your feet on the ground. Your arms and head will not touch the ground any further. Your upper body will be pulled up with your arms stretched out while your legs remain at an angle. Return to the starting position.

7. Jackknife exercise for the advanced – The same exercise as before, except that you will add dumbbells or at home you can also used full water bottles.

8. Knee lift – Lay on the ground. Stretch your arms out beside your body. Pull your knees towards your head with your feet at an angle. Return to the starting position. Your feet will not touch the ground during this exercise.

9. Scissor kicks – lay on the ground with your arms stretched out beside your body. Stretch your legs and lift them off the ground in an alternating motion. It looks like a scissor when you lift and lower your legs. Don't touch the ground and don't forget to breathe.

10. Alternating leg pull – lay on the ground, stretch your arms out beside your body. Stretch your legs and lift them off the ground. Alternate by pulling each knee towards your chest. Return into the starting position. Always keep your legs off the ground. .

11. Fingertips to your toes – lay on the ground stretch your arms towards the ceiling. Stretch your legs towards the ceiling. You're your upper body and try to touch your toes with your fingertips. Lower your body back to the ground. Your arms and legs remain up in the air at all times.

12. Fingertips to your toes with weights – Exactly the same as above. You will take a long bell or two dumbbells to increase the difficulty. At home you can also use two water bottles.

13. Lower abs variation 1 – lie down on a bench and attach the weight to your ankles. Your head will not touch the bench and your legs are placed on the bench in an

angle. Pull your knees towards your head an return to the starting position.

14. Lower abs variation 2 – lie down on a bench, slightly lift your head. Keep your legs stretched and lift them up a little bit. Attach the weights to your ankles. Pull your legs up towards your head with your knees are an angle. Your legs should not touch the bench at any time.

15. Lower abs variation 3 – as above, lie down on a bench, attach the weights and lift your legs up towards the ceiling. Lower them into the starting position. Do not let your legs touch the bench at any time during the exercise.

16. Lower abs variation 4 – everything like above, except that your legs are being placed on the bench in this exercise.

17. Hip lift variation 2 – lie down on a bench. Lift your legs straight up and lift your hips off the bench at the same time. Keep on raising and lowering your hips.

18. Jackknife exercising your lower abs – attach a weight to your ankles. Lie down on the bench with your legs slightly at an angle. Your upper body is being pulled up

at the same time your knees are being pulled up. Return to the starting position. Your feet can be put down during this exercise.

19. Jackknife exercising your lower abs variation 2 – same as above except that your feet are lifted off the bench the entire time.

20. Leg lift using equipment variation 1 – take your position at the equipment and lift your legs up into a 90 degree angle position. Just like you were sitting on a chair you will stretch your legs into a straight position again. .

21. Leg lift using equipment variation 2 – take your position at the equipment. Pull your legs up at an angle just like sitting on a chair. This is the starting position. Lift your legs up even more and return back to the starting position. .

22. Leg lift using equipment variation 3 – take your position at the equipment. Lift your legs up in a stretched position until they are parallel to the ground. Lower them into the starting position.

23. Leg lift using equipment variation 4 – take your position at the equipment. Stretch your legs in a horizontal position lifting them up and down.

24. Leg lift on a bar – hang yourself on to a bar with your legs stretched out keep pulling your knees up and down into the starting position.

25. Leg lift on a bar variation 2 – hang yourself on a bar with your legs stretched out. Pull yourself up into a horizontal position, which means parallel to the ground and return to the starting position.

Lateral abdominal exercises

Whether at home or in the gym, there is something for everyone. Most important is the right way of exercising. Following your eexercise options:

1. Stretching your upper body – lay down on the floor. Lift your legs as if you were sitting on a chair and cross them at ankle height. Lift your upper body off the ground, just enough so that the shoulders and part of the shoulder blades are off the ground. Put your palms on your temples. This is the starting position. Now rotate your body alternating to the right and to the left. Exercise slowly and focused.

2. Lateral crunch– Lay on the ground. Palms at the height of your temple and keep your legs on the ground at an angle. Then put the ankle of one foot on top of the knee of the other leg. Pull your upper body up in a lateral motion. Right elbow to your left knee. Your head will not touch the ground during this exercise. After a few repetitions you can alternate directions by pulling the left elbow to the right knee.

3. Lateral lift of the legs – support yourself on the ground with one lower arm and one foot. Lift your body so it does not touch the ground anymore. Your other arm is stretched out on top of your body. The upper leg is pulled up and then stretched out again. After a few repetitions switch sides. Don't forget to breathe.

4. Lateral hip lift – Lay on your side. Cross your arms over your chest. Stretch your legs. Lift up your hips together with your legs. Your legs will not be placed on the ground during this exercise.

5. Lateral sit ups variation 1 – Lay on the ground with your legs angled, and your palms on your temples. Now lift your upper body as if you would want to touch your left

knee with your right elbow. Then switch to left elbow towards right knee.

6. Lateral sit ups variation 2 – similar to the above, except that your elbows will switch without lowering your upper body. Starting position, you're your upper body, left elbow to the right knee, stay up and bring your right elbow to your left knee.

7. Lateral sit ups variation 3 – Start from the following position: Pull your upper body up , your hands will be on your chest to hold the weight, angle your legs against a wall (so you won;t slide forward). Your upper body will stay in the same position and only move from left to right and vice versa.

8. Rotate your upper body while sitting down – Sit upright on a bench. Place one long bar behind your head slightly below the neck. Hold the long bell with your hands. Now rotate your body from right to left and vice versa.

9. Rotate your upper body standing up – this exercise is the same as above, except that you stand up with your feet shoulder width apart.

1. Lateral lifting and dipping of you upper body with a long bell - stand shoulder width apart and hold the long bell behind your head slightly below the neck. Tilt sideways as if you would like to touch the outside of your knee with the long bell. Stand upright again and repeat the same to the other side.

11. Lateral dip with your upper body using a long bell – stand shoulder width apart. One hand behind your head, the other stretched out beside your body. This is the hand you hold the long bell with as additional weight. Dip towards the floor and return to the starting position. After a few repetitions switch sides.

12. Lift your upper body variation 1 – place yourself on to of the equipment you want to use and bend your upper body forward towards the ground with your palms on your temples. Now lift your upper body up sideways, as if you wanted to look at your opposite heel. Return to the starting position. Lift your body up again as if you wanted to look at your other heel. You will stress your other side. Return to your starting position and repeat the exercise alternating sides a few times. This also strengthens your back

13. Lifting your upper body variation 2 – Start from the same position as above. Now lift your upper body as if you wanted to look at one hell then the other. Then return to the starting position.

Workout plan

It is advisable to set up a daily workout plan where every muscle group will be exercised at least once. If you don't have enough time, then you should dedicate one work out to your arms, the next one to your legs, then your stomach, next your back etc. Always work one muscle group.

This will keep a balance and you will see some result very soon.

Following some sample workout plans:

1. *First variation*

   Monday, Wednesday, and Friday: one exercise each from the following groups: arms, shoulders, chest, back, legs. Put some more emphasis on the stomach, one exercise for each abdominal muscle group. After you work out you need to stretch and before you need to warm up, for example with a jump rope.

   Tuesday and Thursday: cardiovascular training

2. *Second variation*

   Monday, Wednesday, and Friday: Cardiovascular training, alternate between swimming, power walking, bicycling, or any other exercise of your choice.

3. *Third variation*

   Monday, Wednesday, and Friday: warm up with cardio, just a little shorter – about 15 minutes. Afterwards full body exercise, for each muscle group one set, and don't forget to stretch at the end.

   It is very important to always have different variations when you are working out. You should not use the same training plan for more than four weeks. However, due to all the varieties of the exercises it's not even possible that your workout sessions will be monotonous and boring. The variations will bring the excitement to your workout.

Working out after giving birth

Don't worry; you will get back in shape after giving birth. Like everything this will take some time. You need to adapt to the total change to your lifestyle. But regress exercises are important for your body.

You will be able to prevent a uterine prolapse and urinary incontinence. However, immediately after childbirth it is not advisable to strain yourself with working out. After all it has just shown an incredible performance. You should only start working out normal about 6-8 weeks after your pregnancy.

Before this you should only try to do light exercises for the pelvic floor and lateral abdominals. Everything else would be too much, and if you do nothing at all it is too little. Integrate some soft exercises for the pelvic floor and the lateral abdominals in your new daily routine.

As soon as your doctor is giving you the green light you can start with your daily pre-pregnancy workout plan. While you are pregnant you should not exercise too much and get exhausted. During that time you should be cautious and careful.

Don't worry, if you had a toned body before your body you will be back in shape very soon.

You want to embark on a new path after your pregnancy and giving birth. A six pack ab should not be a dream. Healthy eating habits, exercise and a good workout plan and you will look better than before. You can be mobile outdoors even with your baby.

Stretching

Stretching is very important in sports and working out. Muscles are continuously contracted and tightened and get tense over time. In order to bring them back to their normal form we have to stretch them.

Building muscle will also bring you better results. But most important is that you will stay fit and prevent the shortening of any muscle. Following some basic stretching exercises:

1.   Inside leg – put your legs apart, about three to four times the shoulder width. Keep one leg stretched out while you bend the other one. Lower your pelvis as far as

possible towards the ground. You will feel the stretching on the inside of your leg. Switch and do the same exercise with your other leg. By no means just swing back and forth.

2.   Chest muscle – kneel on the floor, put your arms in front of you. And try to touch the floor with your chest.

3.   Arm muscles – let one arm dangle behind your head towards the shoulder blades. Grab your elbow with the other hand and push down slowly. Alternate between arms.

4.   Hip flexor – Get to the quadruped stand and keep your back straight. Make a cat's back and go back to the starting position.

5.   Stretch your butt lying down – lay on your back, stretch your arms in front of you. Your legs are stretched out. Pull your leg up over the other one at a 90 degree angle and push towards the ground.

6.   Lower arms – stand shoulder width apart. Stretch your arms and pull the fingers of the stretched arm up wards with your other hand.

2.   Thighs – One knee on the floor. The other one is standing on the ground at an angle. Take the ankle of the kneeling leg and pull it back towards your back.

8.   Calves, legs, and buttocks – sit on the floor and stretch both legs. Pull one leg up towards your body with your sole against the other thigh. Grab the sole of the leg which is stretched out and pull your upper body towards your knee.

9.   Hamstrings – lay on the floor with both legs stretched out. Lift one leg and grab it with both hands to pull it closer towards your body.

2. Thigh – stand upright and touch your buttocks with the sole of your foot, grab your ankle with one hand and try to stretch it further.

11. Shoulders – stand straight. Gerade hinstellen. Put your palm on the opposite shoulder. Grab your elbow with the other hand and pull it towards your body.

12. Upper Back – stand shoulder width apart. Bend your upper torso to the side stretching it out.

13. Abdominal muscles – lay on the ground on your stomach. Put your arms beside your chest. Lift your upper body up, tilting you're your head in order to achieve even better stretching.

Summary – Checklists

MOTIVATION

Set yourself a goal – a clear goal will help

Building abdominal muscles

Losing weight

Building muscle mass

Losing weight

Look more attractive

Increase self confidence

Improve your health

*Break down your main goal into milestones –
it is much more motivating if you break down
your main goal into smaller milestones. It is
important to stay realistic. For example: work
out three times a week, eat more fruit, and
lose 6 pounds...*

1. Step   -

_____

_____

2. Step   -

_____

_____

3. Step   -

_____

_____

4. Step   -

_____

_____

5. Step   -

_____

_____

6. Step

_____

____

Reward yourself for every goal you reach - rewards are important, fulfill small wishes you have (now work out pants, fitness machine...).

1. Reward   -

_____

—

2. Reward   -

_____

—

3. Reward   -

_____

—

4. Reward   -

_____

—

5. Reward   -

_____

—

6. Reward   -

_____

—

Before and after photo – take a photo of yourself and place it in a spot where you are always able to see it. Think about the goal you want to accomplish. After you have reached your goal take another photo and place it right beside the first one. This will avoid the jojo effect and you will keep paying attention to your weight.

Success Diary – keep a success diary. Write down and document your success. Write down your weight, BMEI and your measurements. It would be best one weekly basis. With your success dairy you can measure your success and it does help a lot to conquer your inner karma.

Positive Thinking or wishful thinking – just imagine all eyes on you because of your perfect six pack. Imagine your favorite scenario right in front of your eyes once a day, the best time is before you go to sleep. It is well worth it to keep on going for this fantastic goal. Describe in a few sentences what this scenario should look like.

_____

_____

_____

_____

_____

_____

_____

_____

_____

_____

_____

_____

_____

_____

Your weaker self – Just because the great feeling you described about you need to conquer your inner weaker self. It's not worth listening to. It will only bring you down. Your goal is to have a better, easier, and more fulfilled life. Keep on going. Write down how you would feel if you would let your weaker self get the best of you.

_____

_____

_____

_____

_____

_____

_____

_____

_____

_____

_____

Consequent work out – it is important for your body and for our well-being. If you won't work out you will feel bad. Work out on a steady basis and you will feel great. You will feel stronger and feel like on clouds. What will you lose if you give up?

_____

_____

_____

_____

_____

_____

_____

Working out together is easier – do you have a friend who could join you? Even better! You can motivate and pull each other up. Besides this you are less likely to give up as you have someone watching you. Keep on working out until you reach your goal.

SUCCESS DIARY

Work   out
method:_____

Month:_____

Work out rhythm:

Monday - duration_____ min

Tuesday – duration _____ min

Wednesday – duration _____ min

Thursday – duration _____ min

Friday – duration _____ min

Saturday – duration _____ min

Sunday – duration _____ min

Measurements	Week	Week	Week	Week
Height				
Weight				
BMI				

You can add additional measurements in the blank fields, such as stomach, upper arm left, upper arm right, etc..... whatever you would like to pay attention to.

Work Out

Setting goals – in order to reach a better and faster success it is very important to set yourself a goal (I know we already went over this). You will reach your goal faster with some pressure (which means it is best to set yourself a final date).

1. Goal _____

   Date:_____

2. Goal _____

   Date:_____

3. Goal _____

   Date:_____

4. Goal _____

   Date:_____

5. Goal _____

   Date:_____

6. Goal _____

   Date:_____

Where would you like to work out? – You will have a variety of equipment in a fitness studio; however, you can work out in your home without driving or any cost involved...

At home

Fitness Center

A plan for the entire body – if you are a beginner you should train your entire body for the initial period (2-3 months). It will improve your strength and familiarizes your body with the strain. For your strength training it is very important to choose your weights so you can accomplish 12 – 15 repetitions.

1. Month – Weight:_____
   Exercise:_____

   _____

2. Month – Weight:_____
   Exercise:_____

   _____

3. Month – Weight:_____
   Exercise:_____

   _____

Weights and weight bench – with a weight bench, barbell, dumbbell and the right weight you will be perfectly equipped at home. You won't have to buy this if you intend to go to a fitness studio.

Setting up a work out plan – this plan is just as important as setting a goal. Organization is half the battle. You will need a „main thread" you can lean on in order to stay on track working out. Write down a plan.

_____

_____

_____

_____

_____

_____

_____

_____

_____

Circuit training – circuit training is a training unit which can be repeated several times. The training unit can contain one or more exercises which will be repeated about 12 – 15 times. During the first week you should accomplish one training unit, after this you can increase to two, three, or even four units according to your progress.

Exercises for one training unit:

_____

_____

_____

_____

Do it right! – The result will not be accomplished because you exercise fast or from the number of repeats. Exercises should be done at a slower pace, but using every muscle. This will bring you the best result you're your abdominal muscles will tighten.

***The complete abdominal muscle work out* –** it is very important to work out all five areas, one exercise for each

1. Exercise – lower abdominal muscle:

   _____

2. Exercise – upper abdominal muscle:

   _____

3. Exercise – side abdominal muscle:

   _____

4. Exercise – lateral abdominal muscle:

   _____

5. Exercise – lower back:

   _____

It is important to change your routine – as already mentioned above you should practice one unit per abdominal muscle group. To be more successful it is best to interchange the units with all the other muscles groups.

First change in routine:

1. Exercise – lower abdominal muscle:

_____

2. Exercise – upper abdominal muscle:

_____

3. Exercise – side abdominal muscle:

_____

4. Exercise – lateral abdominal muscle:

_____

5. Exercise – lower back:

_____

Second change of routine:

1. Exercise – lower abdominal muscle:

_____

2. Exercise – upper abdominal muscle:

_____

3. Exercise – side abdominal muscle:

_____

4. Exercise – lateral abdominal muscle:

_____

5. Exercise – lower back:

_____

Working out has to be fun – everything that is fun brings much faster results. Weight training also helps to relieve stress. You should feel happier and more energized after each work out.

WORK OUT PLAN

Goal – as always, it is most important to keep your eyes on your goal. Without a goal you will just wander about. Goals are individual for everyone. Perhaps you would like to be attractive, target strengthening, lose weight, and improve your stamina....

1. Goal:

_____

_____

Reaching your goal – you are in control of the road that leads to your goal , as widely known: „Many roads lead to Rome".

1. Work   out   method:

_____
2. Work   out   location:

_____

____

Self-Assessment – to keep a healthy overview you have to assess yourself: what are you able to do already, where are your problem areas....having a great feeling about being successful you should write down your weight and how you are feeling.

_____

_____

_____

_____

_____

_____

_____

_____

Define your main goal – even if the entire body should be worked out once a week, you can still define a focal point. Maybe you would still like to work out your back, shoulders or abs a little more.

1. Main   goal:

_____

Planning your workout – here you will determine how often and how long you will work out. Important! Muscles only grow and regenerate themselves after a recovery phase. This time period is about 24 – 48 hours after each work out. Because of this it is recommended to split up your work out. You certainly can set up working out your entire body, but you need to make sure to have a day of recovery.

1.

Monday:_____

—

2.

Tuesday:_____

—

3.

Wednesday:_____

—

4. Thursday:_____

5.

Friday:_____

 —

6.

Saturday:_____

 —

7.

Sunday:_____

 —

8.

Monday:_____

 —

9.

Tuesday:_____

 —

Work out time schedule – a work out session always consists of three phases: warm up, main work out, cool down. Warm up and cool down together should be equivalent of the time for the work out. For example: work out session of 60 minutes would be divided as following: 15 minutes warm up, 30 minutes main work out, 15 minutes cool down, which consists mainly of stretching.

1. Work out session: _____ Minutes
2. Warm up: _____ Minutes
3. Main work out: _____ Minutes
4. Cool down, stretching: _____ Minutes

Workout regimen – it is very important to include different exercises in your work out plan. You should do pushing, pulling and isometric exercises.

1. Pushing exercise:

_____

_____

_____

2. Pulling exercise:

_____

_____

_____

3. Isometric exercise:

_____

_____

_____

4. Various exercises:

_____

_____

_____

Setting up your workout plan – it is important to develop a system for your work out plan. You either start with the larger muscles groups, and then move to the smaller ones, or vice versa.

Changing your work out plan – in order to really stimulate your muscles you should change up your work out plan. Certainly you should not change anything after two days, but after about 3 month of working out continuously.

1. Work   out   starting   date:

   _____

2. First   date   of   changing   work   out   plan:

   _____

3. Second   date   of   changing   work   out   plan:

   _____

Working out has to be fun   – everything which is fun will bring much quicker results. Weight training will also reduce stress. You will feel happier and more energized after each work out.

NUTRITION

Thoughts about your nutrition – how do you feed yourself? Is your nutrition dominated by pre-packaged foods, or healthy and balanced? Do you keep a diet which focuses on building muscles?

Changing your eating habits and your diet – familiarize yourself with the basics of the best diet. What should I eat? How often should I eat? For example, it is better to have 5-6 smaller meals than eating 2-3 big meals per day.

Fat burning foods – you will need a diet with nutrition that constantly focuses on burning fat, but at the same time it should give you all the important nutrients and proteins you need.

5-6 meals a day – balancing your energy is a very valuable concept. It means to structure your meals the best way. Snacks should be taken 2 hours prior to main meals. This way you will avoid cravings and the metabolism burns stored fat much quicker.

Whole grain products – are better than wheat products. They are made of more complex and longer carbohydrates. Try to avoid eating glucose syrup, trans fat, saturated fat, and modified starches

Plenty of fluids – as with everything else you should not choose any kind of fluids which are too high in sugar content (Coke, Lemonade), as well as staying away from water which contains too much sodium. It is recommended to drink about 3-4 liters per day.

Stop your cravings – when you switch your diet you will see signs of withdrawal. Your body will miss sweets the most. In order to avoid cravings it helps to brush your teeth, drink a glass of water, chew some gum, or simply eat some fruit.

Setting up a diet plan – the best way is to set up a weekly or two week diet plan. This way you will have an overview and you can make sure that you get all the important nutrients you need to have. You should list every daily meal.

One Re-feed Day per week – this day is important because you can eat whatever you like. It will speed up your metabolism and keep it balanced. Besides this it will motivate to keep on going.

Lose your old habits and get new ones – human beings are creatures of habit. In the beginning it will not be so easy to keep up with the new diet plan. However, after some time you will see how this new plan will give you much more energy and zest for life.

DIET PLAN

Basics about nutrition – as nutrition carries a very broad spectrum you should at least get to know the basic knowledge. This will help you with setting up a diet plan.

Calculating caloric requirements – the complete caloric requirements are very important for your overall diet plan. The total caloric consumption consists of the energy needs and the basic metabolic needs. You can find a lot of different calorie calculators on the internet.

Setting your goal – it is important to know what you really want.

Put on weight – consuming more calories than you can use.
Lose weight – consuming less calories then you need.

Setting up your diet plan – you should eat a variety of foods each day, whereas one day should be a re-feed day. You should consume 5-6 meals a day. You should pay attention to which nutrients you consume at what time during the day. Following an example to keep an overview about your diet plan, of course you can always set up your own charts as well

Week 1	Monday	Tuesday	Wednesday	Thursday	Friday	Saturday	Sunday
Meal 1							
Meal 2							
Meal 3							
Meal 4							
Meal 5							
Meal 6							

Week 2	Monday	Tuesday	Wednesday	Thursday	Friday	Saturday	Sunday
Meal 1							
Meal 2							
Meal 3							
Meal 4							
Meal 5							
Meal 6							

One meal every 3 hours – this averages about 5-6 meals a day

1. Morning: long chain whole grain carbohydrates.
2. Breakfast: long chain whole grain carbohydrates with protein.
3. Lunch: long chain whole grain carbohydrates, lean meats, vegetables, and fruit.
4. Before working out: short chain and long chain carbohydrates, easy to digest protein.
5. After working out: 0,7-1g Dextrose per kg body weight with 30-60g easy to digest protein.
6. Diner: low fat Greek yoghurt or tuna fish.

Food product – following some examples for a better overview:

1. Short chain carbohydrates: Marmalade, fruit juices, fruit...
2. Long chain carbohydrates: Whole grain products, whole grain rice, whole grain pasta, whole grain bread, potatoes...

3. Protein: lean meat, fish, turkey breast, low fat yoghurt, cottage cheese, egg whites, milk, protein powder…

4. Fat: fatty fish, olive oil, nuts…

Overall balance calculation – you can calculate the overall balance with a free calorie calculator, for example with a Kaloma calculator . The overall balance will be compared and coordinated with your metabolism. There can be a deviation of +/- 500 Kcal.

Change in diet plan – No matter how good your diet plan may be, it should be changed from time to time as it only contains 5% of all the nutrition.

Enjoy Eating – Keep in mind that the right diet together with the proper work out is the key to a dream body. Still, you have to have fun eating; otherwise it will just create a counter effect. The period of change will be the most difficult one. Afterwards you will be much happier with your new diet plan.

CARDIOVASCLUAR WORK OUT

Cardiovascular workout – is important for the cardiovascular system, as well as the metabolism, which in turn is mandatory for building muscles and burning fat. Another effect will be melting away stored fat. It is recommended to go running about two or three times a week.

Working out in the healthy zone – working out should be within the healthy zone in order to strengthen the cardiovascular system and stimulate burning fat. The healthy zone is between 50 – 60% of the maximum heart frequency. The stress factor should be light to medium and last about 30-40 minutes. um das Herz-Kreislauf-System zu stärken und die Fettverbrennung.

Your own rhythm – each body is unique, What may be too fast for one, might be too slow for the other. You have to find your own speed to find the perfect point to burn fat. You should still be able to have a conversation while you are running. This is a general guideline. If you strain your body too much you will burn glucose and the fat will remain. The effect you wanted to achieve will not happen at all.

Keeping your torso straight – you have to learn how to run. You should keep your torso, neck and head straight, but not stiff. A little hint: focus looking a couple steps ahead of you, this way you will almost have the perfect posture.

Arm posture – the positioning of your arms is important. Your elbows should be at a 90 degree angle, swinging your arms slightly above your waist with your hands open. You should not swing your arms above your chest or below the center of your body.

Feet and steps – it is enough to lift your feet slightly off the ground. Running does not get more effective lifting your feet up to your chin. In the beginning it is best to take smaller steps, and as you get fit your steps will get bigger.

Relaxing it key – a lot of people will clench their teeth, tighten their face frantically, and make a fist... keep checking your body a couple times when you are running. If you feel any tension – relax!

Regularity will bring more energy – running can give you more energy. But this will only be the case if you do it regularly. It will take a couple weeks or even months to feel a change if you have not been working out. Your body will need some time to change and adapt to the changes.

Integrating cardiovascular training in your work out – You do not have to set up an additional work out plan, quite the opposite. You should integrate it into your existing plan.

Fun factor – running can almost turn into meditation. It is the perfect balance to everyday stress. If you combine running with nature you will accomplish a sense of well-being. In any case you should have fun while working out. Otherwise you will not accomplish anything at all. While running through nature you should clearly have your goal in front of your eyes. Try to imagine it as graphic as possible. You can bet on it that you will accomplish it all the sooner.

SIXPACK

Basics for the ideal six pack – without the basics, without a beginning, or an end there is no goal. Once again the most important factors:

1. Optimum nutrition
2. Low body fat index of about 10%
3. Effective work out plan

Lowering your body fat index – this can be accomplished with a well-balanced diet and regular cardiovascular workout. Ideal would be to run or bicycle two or three times a week for 30-50 minutes. This ramps up your metabolism and stored fat will start to melt away to reveal your hidden six pack.

Dietary change – with 5-6 meals per day it is possible to burn more fat. To schedule more meals is healthier and will provide the body with more nutrients than two big meals per day, which will only stress your stomach. A healthy diet has to be planned.

Work out plan – a well thought out work out plan is another basic requirement. It has to fit your individual needs. No matter what, you should work out 2-3 times per week. The work out should include all importnat muscle groups, such as arms, chest, abs, legs,back and shoulders. Cardiovascular workout should be an integral part of your workout routine. Of course you can focus on certain muscle groups in addition to this. But keep in mind that everything needs to be balanced otherwise you will start to look a little bit funny.

Whole body workout – all the muscle groups are connected. In order to accomplish a great result in the shortest amount of time you need to work out your entire body. This is absolutely necessary if you want to get perfect ripped abs. Of course you can target other muscle groups as well, but you should do it with moderation.

Regeneration – the regeneration phase is very important. Without regeneration muscles won't grow bigger. In between work out session you need 24 to 48 hours. It is also very important to sleep an average of 7 to 8 hours.

Working out your abdominal muscles – you should work out your abdominal muscles two or three times a week at the beginning of your work out session. Otherwise you might be too tired and won't perform the exercises correctly. Don't overdo it because the abdominal muscles grow and get stronger during the relaxation phase.

Enough fluids – they are important for the metabolism and support burning fat. Three liters of fluids are necessary each day. If you work out more you should also drink more.

Nutritional rules – are necessary to make your hidden six pack visible. Even later on nutrition is a vital part as you could lose the abs you just worked so hard on and they will be back to hiding under a layer of fat.

Having fun working out – is the key point, otherwise you will not succeed. You won't see a six pack overnight, it will take time. Every time you work out you relief stress and are happier, as long as you are having fun.

I hope that I was able to help you getting one step closer to your goal with this self-help book, and hope that you will reach all your goals and live a richer life.

Yours, Jörg Weber

P.S. Did you read my first book?

Burning belly fat or the truth about six pack abs – how you can burn your stomach fat and build stomach muscles in 30 minutes.

Would you like to burn your Stomach fat? Would you like to find out the truth about stomach muscles? Then this book is absolutely perfect for you.

This is what you will read:

- How to build stomach muscles in 30 minutes

- Why a flat stomach is better for your body

- Why burning fat is essential for your life

- Why your stomach muscles are good for your back

- 14 rumors about burning fat and a flat stomach and of course the truth about them

- Whether health food or labeled products are really healthy

- Talk about fab diets

- Are there any foods you can eat to lose weight?

- How about weight loss pills?

- Benefits of sit ups and push-ups

- Can you get big by lifting weights?

- Is endurance work out really necessary?

- What is the story behind carbs?

- Do you have to cut out fat completely from your diet?

- What is the impact on your body when you lose weight too fast?

- Can you get a flat stomach in 5 easy steps?

- Does targeted exercise work for certain body areas?

- How much exercise do you really need?

- What is healthy eating anyway?

- How big can your serving size be?

- How do you really lose weight?

- Aides and support you really need?

- How to burn fat the right way?

- Everything about toned and defined stomach muscles

- Why it does not help to just do sit ups

- How about stomach exercising equipment on TV?

- Which exercises are the best for your stomach muscles?

- How to maintain the goals you have reached

Buy now http://www.amazon.com/Burning-Belly-Truth-about-ebook/dp/B007GPT404/